'Seeing your posts definitely changed my mindset about good and bad foods and it helped me a lot during my battle to recover from anorexia as it really helped me get over my "fear foods".' Ariane, UK

'I struggled a lot with my relationship with food and your page helped immensely with my fear of "unhealthy" foods. I feel so much better and allow myself treats in moderation.' Lara, Germany

'I always enjoy the gym, but I was careless with my calories and as a result, was not in a deficit but actually gaining weight. What I have enjoyed is sitting at home, enjoying a bar of chocolate, or ordering a pizza, eating it and not feeling guilty because I had factored it in. And that's massively down to you and your content. So thanks!' Steve, UK

'Because of you, and the individuals within the Fitness Chef community group, I feel like I've completely taken control and ownership of my life and relationship with food...Having read both your books, and after cooking a few of your meals, I feel empowered!' Erin, Scotland

LOSE
WEIGHT
WITHOUT LOSING
YOUR MIND

Graeme Tomlinson

THE FITNESS CHEF

LOSE WEIGHT WITHOUT LOSING YOUR MIND

Free yourself from diet myths & food guilt

EBURY
PRESS

CONTENTS

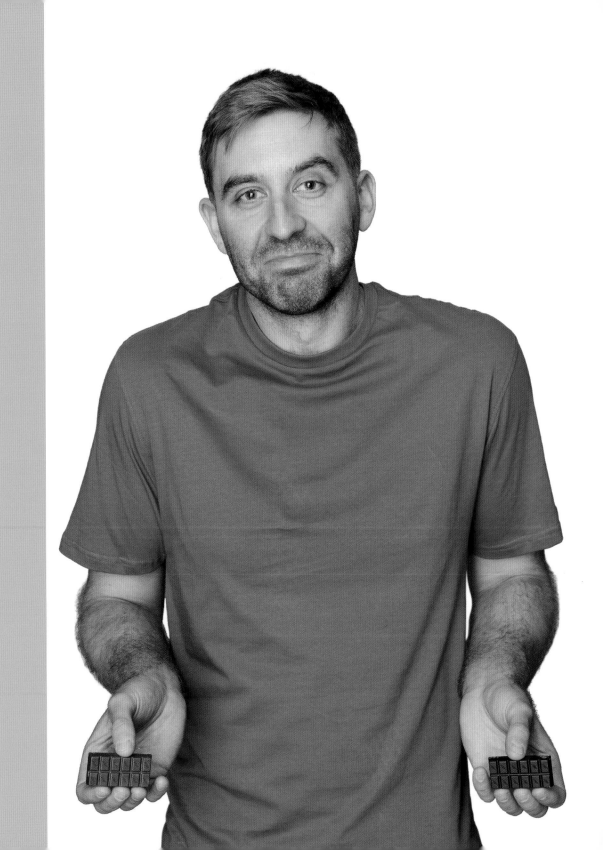

INTRODUCTION

Think you need to suffer to lose weight?
Get ready to change your mind.

In January 2021, I watched a popular diet show on how to lose weight. The presenters selected what they believed to be the best diets for weight loss. One contestant was given the same diet that a world-famous singer used to lose a staggering 7 stone. One was given a diet limited to coffee, water and smoothies. Another was restricted to a gluten- and dairy-free diet high in antioxidants, with carbs forbidden after 4pm. Among the other weight-loss interventions were 24-hour fasts twice a week, meaning no solid food for days at a time, and a diet that promised to be effective not only for weight loss but...wait for it... also for looking like a pop star. Perhaps the strangest were the diet that instructed participants to avoid so-called 'stupid' foods such as dairy, sugar and processed foods, and 'the chocolate diet' where the dieter would be eating 'good' chocolate instead of 'bad' chocolate.

The show also explored methods of appetite suppression. Changing the colour of food to blue was advocated as a way to stop overeating, on account of the blue reminding us of mould or fungus and making us so repulsed that we wouldn't feel hungry any more. Blue spectacles and magic food mirrors, plates and bowls that made a serving of food look larger than it was were said to work by giving the illusion that a slice of cake was double the size. We would then believe we were eating more than we actually were. Which left me wondering who was kidding who.

It's important to maintain your perspective when you're watching TV and remember that the point is to entertain. It would be boring to see easy, consistent weight loss over time. Unsurprisingly the show emphasized the struggles the participants endured on their diets. After days of being restricted to eating foods he loathed, one contestant caved in: 'My wife has only gone and cooked sausage, mash and onions with gravy... and I've gotta tell ya, I'm actually gonna eat it!' Others talked of cravings for foods they enjoyed but said they would feel too guilty and ashamed to eat now. To fit the thrills, spills, cliffhangers and happy endings that TV demands, in the end, after all the torture, all participants lost weight. However, all professed to detesting their diets so much that they would be abandoning them as soon as the show was over.

While the contestants lost weight during the show, given that they couldn't stand continuing their diets, what were they supposed to do afterwards to avoid regaining the weight? More 24-hour fasts? More coffee diets? Always colour their food blue? The impression they and the viewers were left with was that losing weight is only possible by cutting out most, if not all, of the foods you enjoy, and that weight loss is synonymous with misery. These extreme diets only offered weight-loss solutions that focused on strictly eliminating foods rather than including foods to enjoy, and they left no flexibility – no option for still leading a good life. What's the point of adopting a diet that means to be your desired size you have to be miserable? Or if it's short-term misery, once you have reached your weight-loss goal, what do you do to happily maintain your new weight?

Amongst the elaborate descriptions of each diet given by the TV presenters there was not one mention of the simplest but most important piece of advice for anyone wanting to lose weight:

If you want to lose body fat, you must be in a calorie deficit, irrespective of the food you choose or the time you eat it.

A calorie deficit = burning more calories than you consume.

This is proven by scientific evidence from around the world. It means that whatever diet the contestants were on, they could only lose weight if they consumed fewer calories than they expended over time. There is no good evidence that suggests the contestants lost body fat because they banned dairy and sugar, ate antioxidants and special types of chocolate, or ate at specific times of the day. Though they were told certain foods were 'fat-burning' or 'fat-causing', they lost body fat because they were in a state of caloric deficit, regardless of the type of food they ate. It's unclear whether they knew this as they were grinding through their tortuous diets. You'd think a reputable TV channel with

> To lose body fat, you must be in a calorie deficit.

a team of producers may have taken the responsible step of pointing out this essential fact to their trusting audience, drawn to a programme that promised a way to lose weight. But the advice was to try a few unsustainable, idiosyncratic eating routines and marketing ideas utterly irrelevant to this key underlying principle. It's the number of calories in vs calories out that defines the amount of body fat you have. Are there other important factors to consider? Sure. But before thinking about those, you need to understand the basics. When those advising us don't start with the basics, then misinformation and confusion spread, and this is partly why so many diets fail.

After seeing the results apparently achieved by these dieting methods, viewers may be inclined to believe that these unnecessary and unsustainable interventions are the best methods for losing weight. So, to lose weight, you must rip up your existing diet, turn your life upside down, eat foods you don't enjoy, refrain from eating for 24 hours, restrict yourself to liquids only and feel miserably hungry for extended periods. This restrictive approach disregards the enjoyment we deserve to have when we eat. It shows no empathy for the person who wants to lose weight and could affect both their physical and mental health.

Such approaches are not limited to television. They are rife in the fitness industry too. It's like the car salesman trying to convince you that you need that expensive new car. 'This new car will change your life!' It may also mean you need a bigger garage, but hey: you'll have the latest version. The salesman doesn't want you to know that the car you already have is the same as the new one except a bit slower and with fewer additional features that you don't actually need. It will run as smoothly as the new one when it's had a service and will look just as good after a wash and minor repairs. With these small improvements the existing car will fulfil all your requirements with no need for you to spend money on a new car and a larger garage. No upheaval, and a car that will serve you well for many years to come, taking you wherever you want to go.

The dieting industry is big business and diet salespeople are everywhere. Some will say you need to be tough and resilient to lose weight. You have to *really* want it. Then comes the brand-new rigid diet. Some will ask you to pay them large sums of money for their secrets. Cross their palm with silver and they'll share the 'good' foods for weight loss and the 'bad' foods that you must avoid at all costs. Some will tell you that signing up to their slimming club is the golden ticket to sticking to a diet that works.

Over the years, thousands of my followers from all over the world have messaged me saying: 'I've tried every weight-loss diet out there and none of them has worked. I don't know what to do any more... What should I be eating?' My answer is always the same:

Losing body fat long-term is not the result of any specially designed diet with glamorous promises.

It is simply the result of your ability to create a calorie deficit over time, while enjoying as many of your food and lifestyle preferences as possible.

There is a way to lose weight long-term and be happy. You can eat all the foods you enjoy and still succeed. There is a weight-loss diet that works so well you will never need to go on another diet ever again. In this book, I'm going to show you why your mind can be your worst enemy or your most powerful asset. Filling it with facts, focus and joy can deliver the long-term weight-loss diet that will work for you, improve your quality of life and boost your happiness.

But simply telling you that a calorie deficit is required to lose weight and then leaving you to it would not be helpful. That's why this book will mentor you with empathy, help you to discern the myths from evidence-based science and give you simple mental strategies and perspectives to transform what may feel like a challenging journey into a simpler and easier path, moulded for long-term behaviour change.

Fortunately, despite all the misery diets and mental gymnastics available, there exists a much better starting point for your weight-loss journey. It's free of charge and one I think you'll enjoy. It's the diet you already have.

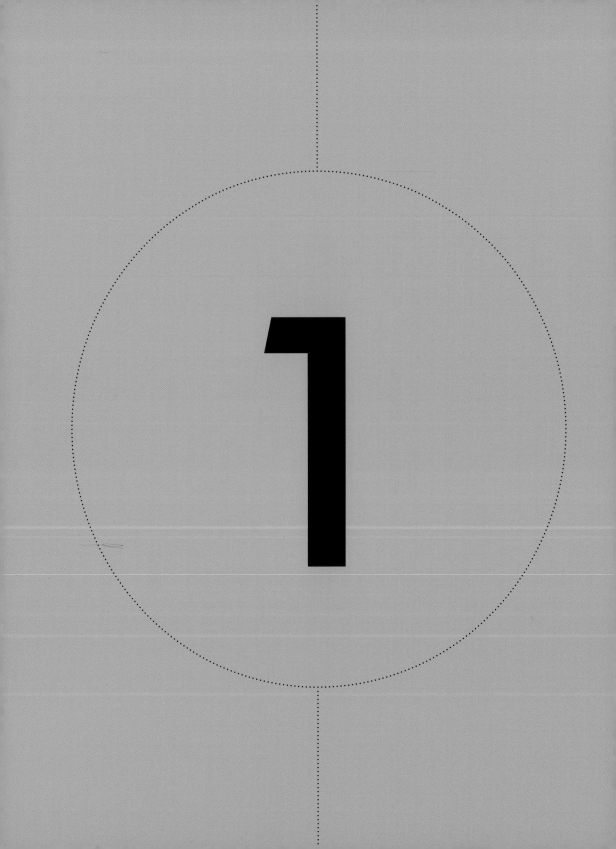

RESET
YOUR FOCUS

WHAT DOES THE 'PERFECT' DIET LOOK LIKE?

According to mainstream media, hundreds of diet books and many medical professionals, to eat well means to focus entirely on eating as many nutritious foods as possible. This picture of nutritional perfection is also demonstrated on social media, with high-profile accounts dedicated to informing people about the health benefits and drawbacks of specific foods.

In the early 1990s, Michael van Straten wrote a book called *Superfoods*. Along with a few others, he is thought to have coined this term, branding a small selection of foods nutritionally superior to others. Many authors, including doctors and registered dietitians, still use this term in cookbooks and diet plans. However, the problem lies in that by placing certain foods on pedestals of perfection, you inadvertently label other foods sub-par.

To be 'perfect means' to be free from faults or defects, to be absolute or complete. It is a term we use daily to describe things we believe to be 'as good as they can be'. If you switch on your TV and grin and bear the adverts, you'll hear the word 'perfect' used to describe products that promise to deliver the very best results. The best frying pan ever created. The best possible deal on a last-minute holiday. Or the best way to lose body fat and be healthy.

When it comes to selecting a method to lose weight and eat healthily, time and time again, we are shown the perfect result in an advert designed to convince us to join. Usually, the actors will smile while documenting how great they feel and how much weight they have lost. Because it's exactly what you want to hear. At a glance, if you want to feel great and lose weight, why wouldn't you try this? Who knows, maybe you will enjoy it? But if you've attempted multiple so-called perfect diets and never been successful long-term, why weren't you successful? In a study spanning thousands of overweight adults in the USA who attempted to lose weight for a year, 40 per cent achieved a 5 per cent reduction in bodyweight, while 20 per cent reported a 10 per cent reduction.[1]

This begs the question: why couldn't the remaining 40 per cent lose weight? The research paper stated that the above figures show reasonable numbers of people can lose weight in the short-term, but what happens in the long-term? With statistics such as '95 per cent of diets fail' flouted around willy-nilly, is it that losing body fat and keeping it off is simply impossible? Are we hardwired to be overweight? Or is it that too many of us choose unsustainable methods over and over again? Do we need to pay more attention to the methods and processes used in weight-loss attempts? What about our habits and long-term behaviours? Are our environments conducive to supportive weight-loss outcomes? Above all, what is going on between our ears? Is it our beliefs that hinder us?

THE MAGIC NUMBER 7

In 1956, George Miller of Harvard University wrote a paper entitled 'The magic number 7' in which he argued that we struggle to remember chunks of information if the amount exceeds seven individual pieces at any given time. Later research has shown that our memory is much more fluid, but if we aren't already familiar with pieces of information, they become more challenging to recall than those we are familiar with. For example, consider a combination of numbers you've known since childhood vs a series of long words written in a foreign language. Trying to recall several longer, unfamiliar pieces of information at one time is going to be more difficult, but you'll give it a go, even if you are sure there will be errors. But when the list of unfamiliar words becomes more extensive, it gets even harder, and there's a strong chance you'll give up.

Let's imagine you've seen many adverts showcasing the 'perfect' diet, promising excellent results. Let's call it Diet X. Perhaps you've even heard stories from friends illustrating their outstanding success. But what about the process? The results don't come out of thin air. There must be a catch, right? Yes, there is. If Diet X promises outstanding results but requires you to carry out 100 per cent of the processes to achieve those results, Diet X requires you to be outstanding. Logically, you must be perfect, or you won't have the same success. The product you invest in is only perfect if you're perfect too. If you're not perfect, you fail – and that's on you. Let's hypothesize that Diet X demands that you follow the rules opposite:

Diet X's dubious demands

✗ Eat at specific times of the day.
What they don't tell you is that you will have to restructure your entire day to accommodate this, and you may have to go hungry.

✗ Only eat grass-fed meat.
These meats are expensive and difficult to source, meaning you'll be out of pocket and require extra time to locate them.

✗ Cut out refined sugar.
This statement doesn't justify how difficult this actually is. You will have to check nutrition labels fastidiously and eliminate some of your favourite foods.

✗ Follow a specific exercise regime.
This may mean that you need to buy clothing and possibly equipment as well as finding the time for this.

✗ Stop eating carbs.
This fails to appreciate that most foods aside from meat and dairy contain carbs, meaning eliminating them and finding other foods will be very difficult, but also that you'll likely be removing a lot of foods from your diet. Many of which you enjoy.

✗ Replace carbs with fat.
This leaves you having to take time to research another bunch of foods that fit the bill while being mindful of what type of fat you're eating.

✗ Don't eat after 6pm.
This fails to take into consideration your lifestyle and things such as work and children which mean you can often only eat after 6pm.

✗ Eat superfood X and superfood Y.
This requires time to source these and the extra expense to buy them.

✗ Follow a specific meal plan.
This restricts your freedom to eat anything other than the plan's recipes, banning lots of foods you previously ate and eliminating spontaneous choices.

✗ Take supplements A, B and C.
You need to find these, buy them and then remember to take them every day.

All of a sudden, from being someone who ate a varied diet, with nothing off-limits, that's ten brand-new demands to remember every day. Within these there are sub-demands, too. So that's 30 things to remember to stay on track and get great results. That's a lot of stuff, not to mention constantly fighting yourself to make sure you don't regress to old eating habits not permitted on Diet X. Do some, if not all, of these demands sound both extreme and familiar to you? Do you know why Diet X is demanding this of you in the first place? Why these specific rules?

Later in the book, we'll look at whether any of these demands are relevant to losing weight or improving health, but the sheer volume of upheaval that Diet X (which represents all extreme diets) places on its followers makes it very difficult to stick to. If most of us struggle to recall more than seven pieces of new information, how can we be expected to remember 30 new rules every day on top of everything else going on in our lives?

The most crucial aspect of any dietary change is your ability to stick to it. If your diet is simple, easy to remember and convenient, there's a greater chance you're going to continue with it and more likelihood of achieving the results you want. You may need to tweak a few things here and there but think of it as rearranging a set of single numbers you're already familiar with. Turning your life upside down and trying to recall numerous brand-new behaviours is likely to increase stress and compromise other areas of your life. The chances of sticking to the diet also decrease, especially if you don't know why you're doing it or don't enjoy it.

What are the odds of successfully losing weight? I always imagine the miracle fat-loss diet or slimming club as a casino. They sell you fat loss at favourable odds, meaning each time you try them, the allure of what you could win sucks you in to gamble. Maybe this roll of the dice will finally win me a huge sum of money?! Maybe this fat-loss diet will finally be the one that works...? Have you ever heard the saying, 'the house always wins'? While you may experience some positive results initially, over time the more you gamble, the more money you lose. So, what do you need to do to avoid the weight-loss gamble? If being perfect doesn't work, then what does?

THE CASINO OF DIETS

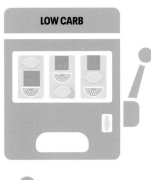

LOW CARB

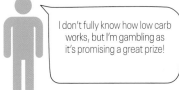

I don't fully know how low carb works, but I'm gambling as it's promising a great prize!

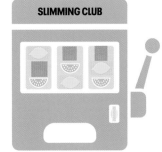

SLIMMING CLUB

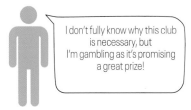

I don't fully know why this club is necessary, but I'm gambling as it's promising a great prize!

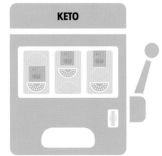

KETO

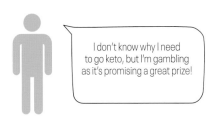

I don't know why I need to go keto, but I'm gambling as it's promising a great prize!

WHAT TO FOCUS ON
FIRST AND FOREMOST

Before embarking on your journey to reduce body fat, you need to know how you are going to get there, and the only scientifically proven way to get there is by creating a calorie deficit.

A calorie is a unit of measurement used to count energy. A deficit just means a shortfall in the amount that's needed.

If you spend more money than you earn ⟶ you create a financial deficit = you lose money

If you spend more calories than you consume ⟶ you create a calorie deficit = fat loss

You can create a calorie deficit in two ways:

1. Reduce the calories you consume

2. Increase the energy you expend

You can also do both simultaneously.

WHAT IS CALORIES IN
VS CALORIES OUT?

CALORIES CONSUMED	CALORIES BURNED

You maintain your weight by consuming and burning approximately the same amount of calories, over time

CALORIES CONSUMED	CALORIES BURNED

You gain weight by consuming more calories than you burn, over time (calorie surplus)

CALORIES CONSUMED	CALORIES BURNED

You lose weight by consuming fewer calories than you burn, over time (calorie deficit)

Calories and energy are effectively the same thing. The amount of energy you consume compared to the amount of energy you burn defines how much body fat you have.

If you consume more calories than you burn
⟶ you store more body fat

If you consume and burn roughly the same number of calories
⟶ you maintain consistent levels of body fat

If you consume fewer calories than you burn
⟶ you reduce your body fat

WEIGHT-LOSS
DIET NOISE

UNDERSTANDING
A CALORIE DEFICIT

It's not about calories!!

Your metabolism is broken

Juice detox!

It's about insulin!!

Don't eat carbs!

Eat as many 'free' foods as you like!

?!?!

Skip breafast!

Go keto!

Count chemicals, not calories

Fasting

Eat breakfast

Don't eat after 6pm

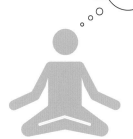

My mindset is clear, allowing me to give more of myself to other aspects of my life

Eating fewer calories than I burn over time results in fat loss – **all the other stuff doesn't matter**

The calorie deficit is not a diet method invented by me or by anybody else, it is human physiology. Whenever you read, see or hear that you need to cut carbs, ban specific foods or eat at certain times, just refocus on this scientifically supported method. Losing body fat will always boil down to being in a state of calorie deficit. Start with this fundamental scientific truth and you'll drown out a hefty chunk of fat-loss misinformation.

Think of it like this: consuming calories does not necessarily result in weight gain or weight loss. You are simply consuming units of energy. But these units of energy add up to define your weight. Eating 2,200 calories per day isn't a problem if you burn more than 2,200 calories. But if you only burn 2,000 calories, you won't lose fat. It's a numbers game.

SUSTAINABILITY IS JUST AS IMPORTANT AS A CALORIE DEFICIT

Understanding that you require a calorie deficit to lose fat is essential. But not as crucial as your adherence to it. Your ability to stick to a calorie deficit, on average, over long periods is key to long-term weight loss. The fat you want to lose didn't appear overnight. It is the result of you having created a calorie surplus over time. In the same way, fat loss won't occur overnight. It will be the result of creating a calorie deficit over time. This doesn't mean you must make sure you're in a calorie deficit every single hour of every single day. It just means on average. We'll discuss this in more detail later in the book.

CONSIDERATIONS
BEFORE STARTING
YOUR WEIGHT-LOSS
JOURNEY

YOUR MOTIVE

Why do you want to lose body fat?
Will it improve your happiness and overall health?
If not, don't do it.

YOUR BELIEF SYSTEM

Understanding that a calorie deficit results in fat loss.

YOUR ACTIONS

Making sure that your behaviours support consuming
fewer calories than you burn, thus adhering to a calorie deficit.

YOUR ENVIRONMENT

Are you putting yourself in situations and surrounding yourself
with people that support or undermine your goal?

YOUR HAPPINESS

How sustainable are your actions and habits over time,
and how much pleasure do you get from them?

BEING REALISTIC

Do you accept that so-called perfection has nothing to do with losing body fat?

TIME

Whatever your motivations, are you prepared
to accept that weight loss takes significant time?

SETTING THE PACE
OF YOUR CALORIE DEFICIT

You know a calorie deficit is the route you need to take, but how fast should you go? A large deficit will result in greater fat loss over a shorter time, but will it be sustainable? Too small a deficit will result in much less fat loss, meaning you may not achieve the desired results at all. So, what's the sweet spot?

Well, let's look at an example. Sally can maintain her current weight by eating 2,200 calories per day. She could reduce this figure by one calorie to eat 2,199 calories per day or by 2,200 to eat 0 calories per day – both represent a calorie deficit, but the difference is enormous. So by how much should Sally reduce her calories?

Research shows that most adults store up to 100,000 calories from body fat at any given time. This means we could technically live for weeks without eating. But this is obviously not advised. After just a few hours without energy, our physical capabilities begin to diminish. Even when sedentary, our bodies constantly burn energy stores, carrying out a whole host of physiological regenerations. Thus, we still experience hunger cues to replenish lost energy stores. Ghrelin is the hunger hormone that reminds us to keep adding calories to fuel and maintain our energy levels for optimal body function. Leptin is the hunger hormone that tells us when we are full and, for the time being, our bodies will not need more calories to improve function.

Suppose Sally reduced her calories from 2,200 to 2,199 and stuck to it religiously. This is not anywhere near enough to result in significant fat loss over 50 years, let alone five months. What if Sally reduced her calories from 2,200 to 0 and stuck to it? She'd be in a huge calorie deficit, but she'd eventually die unless she ate.

These are two extreme examples. But the point is: even if fat loss is your aim, you still require significant amounts of energy to support your bodily systems and avoid extreme hunger. Let's go back to Sally. The answer is actually dependent on many aspects of Sally's life, including her sex, age, height, weight and activity level. Even factoring in her occupation may be very useful. Doing this helps us see how many calories Sally expends each day (her total daily energy expenditure, or TDEE, see page 40). From here, it's a case of subtracting a chunk of calories to create a deficit that is sustainable and effective.

The Harris-Benedict and Mifflin-St Joer equations are regarded as the most accurate methods used by fitness and medical professionals to determine a sustainable calorie figure for losing, maintaining or gaining weight. Fortunately, you don't need to do any complicated maths. If you head to my website, you can get your free calorie target for your goal in just a few seconds – visit www.fitnesschef.uk.

Sally is 35 years old, 5ft 8in, 75kg and lightly active, meaning she walks around 35,000 steps each week, along with 1–2 light to moderate workouts. According to the Harris-Benedict equation, Sally would require approximately 2,200 calories per day to maintain her current weight – as long as her energy expenditure didn't dramatically change. But to lose fat, Sally's new daily calorie target would be approximately 1,850 calories. This is around a 15 per cent reduction, which creates a significant enough deficit to reduce body fat after a few weeks. It's also a small enough calorie reduction for Sally to sustain. As Sally loses weight and wants to continue losing more weight, she needs to recalculate her calorie target to ensure she's still in a calorie deficit. This is because as Sally loses weight, she will burn fewer calories as her body is smaller. It's that simple.

Many people report initial weight-loss success followed by a plateau where they insist that they're in a calorie deficit, but all progress has stopped, leaving them confused and losing faith in a calorie deficit as a route to weight loss. But this is because although they might believe they are in a calorie deficit, they actually aren't. I'll discuss the reasons for this later in the book (see pages 184–6). But for now, be assured any weight-loss plateau is not the result of a calorie deficit suddenly ceasing to work.

CALORIE COUNTING
TO STAY ON TRACK

Calorie counting is fairly self-explanatory. It is the practice of obtaining the calorie values of foods and drinks to understand how many calories you're consuming. Fortunately, it is a legal requirement for food companies to disclose this as part of the nutrition information on their packaging.

Counting calories does not guarantee that you're in a calorie deficit because you may count inaccurately, and your body always answers to the actual number of calories you consume and expend. But it is the most logical way to understand if you are in a calorie deficit or not. Measuring calories consumed may be prone to slight discrepancies, or food labels can be slightly inaccurate on occasion, but that's no reason to throw this approach out completely. If followed as accurately as possible, calorie counting can be instrumental to weight loss, and crucially, very simple. There are many calorie tracking websites and apps that make this process very easy. To start a free trial with my app, visit www.fitnesschef.uk.

I regularly hear stories from people saying that they tried calorie counting, but it didn't work. Or that they switched from a slimming club to calorie counting and it did. But it isn't the method that defines the outcome; it is the principle. If you don't count the calories you eat, it doesn't necessarily mean you won't create a calorie deficit. Think of it as managing a bank balance. If you're aware of income and expenditure, you're informed about financial decisions that make saving money much more straightforward, with less effort required. If you don't know how many calories you're eating, it's hard to know what portion sizes will support fat loss.

If you consume fewer calories than you burn, you will lose body fat.

As I'll discuss later, many people continue to deny that calories in vs calories out (or calorie balance) is why we lose, maintain or gain fat. Dieting ideologies such as low carb, keto, slimming clubs or intermittent fasting continue to claim that their method works better as a way of losing body fat. Within these diets, some agree that calorie balance is essential but that their way optimizes fat loss. Others flat out deny that calories have anything to do with accumulating or losing body fat. The latter often confuse calorie counting with being the same thing as a calorie deficit. It's not. One is a method that involves tracking calories; the other is a physiological phenomenon that will occur with or without counting calories.

Regardless of whether you choose to count calories, the calories in the food you eat will influence your weight one way or the other. Think of it like having £200 in your bank account and going shopping without checking the price tags on your purchases or even having a rough idea of how much the items cost. Checking the calorie values is just like checking the prices. By checking the calorie values of foods that you buy regularly, you develop a sense of how many calories each food contains and don't need to always keep checking, just as you develop a sense of how much money things cost. This enables you to manage your budget.

If weight loss is your goal, I recommend having an idea of the calorie values of the foods you eat, even if you don't want to track your calories meticulously. Think of it as increasing your awareness and part of the process of nourishing yourself with useful data to help you reach your weight-loss goal. It also helps you to understand portion sizes. Soon, you should be able to eyeball portion sizes that represent specific calorie values. For example, weighing out 50g oats every day for a week should be enough for you to visualize 50g oats so that you no longer need to weigh them. You could also use a sticker or pen to mark a container at the height of different portions and use the marked container as a measure until you don't need it any more.

Your ability to gauge the calories in foods that you eat regularly will serve you well beyond your immediate weight-loss goal, enabling you to maintain your desired weight and enjoy your food, using your judgement to balance calories so you don't regain any weight you lose. Taking a few weeks to familiarize yourself with the calorie values of different portion sizes is empowering and a good investment in your health and happiness. It will put you in control of your weight and free you from the misery of unsustainable diets for the rest of your life. The higher the number of calories in a food, for example peanut butter, which contains around 600 calories per 100g, the more accuracy is required. But foods such as broccoli, which contains just 40 calories per 100g, are so low in calories that you don't need to measure them quite as accurately.

If you start to think that counting calories is too obsessive, take a step back and remind yourself why you're doing it. To understand how many calories you have consumed relative to the amount you need to achieve your weight-loss goal – that's it. Much like saving money for a holiday and checking your bank balance every few days to make sure you're on course to get to your desired destination. While some portray calorie counting as a lifelong draining of psychological resources, you can utilize it as an education, simple enough to remember for life. Like businesses collect data on their customers' preferences to improve sales, understanding and recording calorie values can educate us to make informed choices that support our calorie needs.

BEWARE OF UNDER REPORTING

In a Columbia University study, people claimed they were eating 1,200 calories per day while also reporting that they couldn't lose weight. The data showed that they were consuming 47 per cent more calories than they thought and were burning 51 per cent fewer calories than they claimed.[7] This isn't necessarily a red flag against the usefulness of calorie counting. Still, it does highlight that accurate tracking is important and our memories and assumptions can sometimes fail us.

In the words of the astronomer Galileo: 'Measure what can be measured and make measurable what cannot be measured.' Backed up Lord Kelvin, 'If you cannot measure it, you cannot improve it'. In other words, measuring something makes us focus on it and gives us a starting point and a measure of progress. Without this, we are relying on our fallible memories and assumptions, as seen in the Columbia University study.

I DON'T EAT MUCH
BUT I CAN'T LOSE FAT

IN YOUR HEAD

IN REALITY

210 cal   105 cal   245 cal   245 cal

210 cal   220 cal   220 cal   683 cal

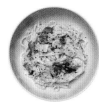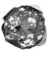

140 cal   390 cal

993 cal

'Not too much...'*

3,661 cal
(aka probably not a calorie deficit)**

*Correction: not much volume, but still consumption of a lot of calories
** This is precisely why tracking calorie intake is useful for fat loss

Why some calorie-tracking apps can cause problems

Many calorie-tracking apps I have seen generate mindset struggles before a single food has been logged. They typically present users with the option to choose between a tough, high-calorie deficit calculated to achieve their weight-loss goal in the shortest time possible or a smaller – more easily achievable – deficit calculated to achieve their weight-loss goal over a longer period. While this isn't the inherent fault of these apps, the option to lose a vast amount of weight over a shorter time understandably appeals to an eager and impatient user, who may not be aware that the gentler calorie deficit offers a greater chance of success due to its sustainability long-term.

When the option is there to lose around 1kg (2–3lb) per week aggressively, it can be just too tempting. It gets selected because users are focused on fast results instead of the long game. Try to focus on following a calorie deficit that you can comfortably sustain and know that this will get you to your weight-loss goal.

1,200 CALORIES A DAY IS NOT THE ANSWER

Users of calorie-tracking apps generally end up with calibrated targets of 800–1,200 calories per day. This is a calorie deficit alright, but for most body sizes, a mighty miserable one that is unlikely to last. You do not have to be constantly hungry to lose weight. You can eat more than 1,200 calories per day and still lose body fat.

Alarmingly, I have noticed a daily target of 1,200 calories becoming a common goal in the online weight-loss community (perhaps related to the apps being used), with many seeing anything above this target as scuppering their progress, but unless you're relatively short and not carrying much body fat – it isn't!

YOUR WEIGHT IS JUST A NUMBER

A slimming club bases your success on your ability to lose vast amounts of weight week by week and hands out praise and prizes to the biggest losers, but weight loss isn't linear – your weight doesn't decrease at a set rate in equal amounts each day – and your bodyweight is made up of more than just fat. Rather than getting caught up in the short-term, viewing weight loss as an average over time is more realistic. Losing an average 225–400g (0.5–1lb) per week over six months is likely to be more sustainable than trying to lose around 1kg (3lb) per week. Each time you step on the scales, that number you see measures your complete biological structure, not just the amount of fat you have. So never let that number determine how you feel about yourself and never let any person reading it to you demoralize you. As long as you adhere to your calorie deficit over time, you will be making progress towards your goal, even when the scales don't change between weigh-ins. I'll talk more about why the number on the scales isn't significant in the short-term later, see page 125. But for now, I recommend focusing on progress photos instead of regularly stepping on the scales. This measuring method lets you see changes, regardless of how much you weigh, and with less pressure.

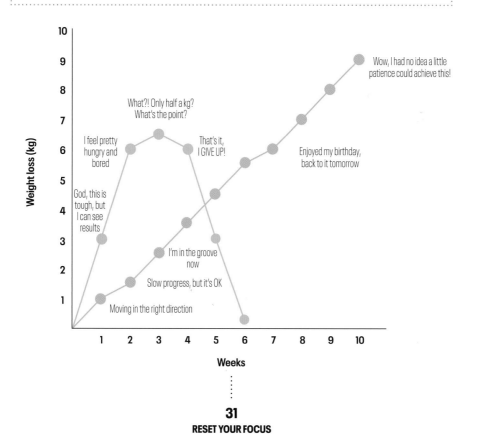

Think weekly,
not daily

The calorie target you get from online calculators gives you a daily figure to aim for. Let's say your target is 2,000 calories per day for fat loss. Over seven days, that equals 14,000 calories. But instead of trying to achieve 2,000 calories every day, what about trying to achieve 14,000 calories across seven days? Spreading your calorie intake across a week ultimately won't change the numbers you have to aim for, but it gives you much more flexibility. You can enjoy calorie-dense social occasions, knowing you can rein back calorie intake across other days to stay on track. If you go over your target one day, you haven't failed. You have the next day to adjust, and what you do next counts most (see page 146). This relaxed mindset also allows you to plan for calorie-dense eating episodes like social occasions by reducing calorie intake the day before or earlier the same day. This flexible strategy is much easier to manage and shows why losing weight doesn't need to be gruelling or require you to unhappily follow regimented daily targets, eating with constant self-discipline. In fact, not adhering to daily targets, aka the opposite of being perfect, may even ultimately result in greater success. Why? Because you have realized this is a game of averages over time, not short-term, constant perfection, making the process more doable and easier to adhere to.

A sports team doesn't win the championship with one victory; they need many individual victories over a long period. The team may lose some matches, but that doesn't mean they'll lose the championship. If the team wins the championship, they simply had more wins than losses. There is no pressure because there's always another opportunity around the corner. Despite having a daily target of 2,000 calories, you can succeed by never eating 2,000 calories in a single day. Why? Because you maintained an average of 2,000 calories per day. To switch to tracking your targets weekly instead of daily, or to do a mixture of both, visit www.fitnesschef.uk and start your free trial.

THE STOP AND THINK HABIT

A typical sales tactic used across multiple industries is creating or highlighting a problem and offering a solution. In most industries, this is very useful. If you have a jacket that isn't waterproof and you often walk in the rain, seeing an advert for a reliable waterproof jacket may be the perfect answer to your problem. What if you'd like to lose weight and a brand-new fat-loss diet is advertised as the solution to your problem? This seems timely and the ideal answer to your goal. But the difference between the waterproof jacket and fat loss is that the first is simple. The jacket is an instant solution, but fat loss is a complex series of physical and mental changes that requires your time and commitment. Despite how much weight the new diet promises you're going to lose, losing weight isn't instant and the solution needs to come from you.

The challenge is to stop and think. Clever advertising shows before and after transformations of people who have supposedly benefited from the diet, but what about the process required to get there? Naturally, we're drawn to the results, which means we're likely to ignore the relevant process, even if it's extreme. Ask: Do I see myself sticking to what is required? Later in the book, I'll talk more in-depth about the benefit of focusing on the process instead of the outcome – hour to hour, day to day, week to week, month to month (see page 139). What happens in these seemingly mundane periods is what will define your success. Your repetition of the process determines your outcome.

There's no such thing as an empty calorie

As we've seen, a calorie is a unit of measurement that measures energy. A gram is a unit of weight that isn't empty. A millilitre is a unit of volume that isn't empty. By the same logic a calorie is a unit of energy that can never be empty. So why do people say things like 'not all calories are created equal' or 'that has empty calories', or even 'a calorie is not a calorie'? Each of these statements suggests that food quality is intrinsically linked to the 'type' of calorie. Well, here's where the confusion lies...

Each food contains calories, and these calories are made of three macronutrients: protein, carbs and fats. Our bodies use calories for every bodily process. They even use calories from the food we eat to digest the food we eat. The number of calories used to digest a particular food depends on its macronutrients because we use more calories digesting some macronutrients than we do others.

Protein = 4 calories per gram
Burns about 25–30 per cent of its calories when it is being digested.
For every 100 calories of protein eaten
➙ 70–75 calories are available to be used as energy or stored as body fat.

Carbs = 4 calories per gram
Burn around 10 per cent of their calories when they are being digested.
For every 100 calories of carbs eaten
➙ around 90 calories are available to be used as energy or stored as body fat.

Fat = 9 calories per gram
Burns around 2 per cent of its calories when it is being digested.
For every 100 calories of fat eaten
➙ 98 calories (virtually all) of them are available to be used as energy or stored as body fat.

This is why high-protein diets are beneficial for anyone looking to lose body fat. As well as burning over a quarter of its calories in the digestion process, protein is filling, and being fuller after eating means

WHY CALORIES ARE CREATED EQUAL
but why macronutrients are created different

Eating 300 calories of
FATS

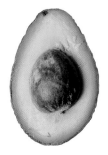

Eating 300 calories of
CARBS

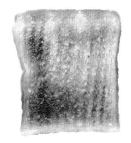

Eating 300 calories of
PROTEIN

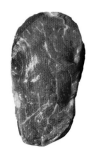

You will burn approximately
2% of these calories during
digestion which = 6 calories

You will burn approximately
10% of these calories during
digestion which = 30 calories

You will burn approximately
25% of these calories during
digestion which = 75 calories

net consumption
294 cal

net consumption
270 cal

net consumption
225 cal

*Net calories consumed may vary depending on the ratio of different macronutrients.
But calories will always remains as equal units of energy.

you're less likely to overeat. Keep eating carbs and fats, but make sure you eat enough protein. Research shows that eating 1–2g protein per kg of bodyweight is beneficial for general health and fat loss. I'll explain the benefits of protein in more detail on page 76.

The term 'empty calories' is usually attributed to foods like cakes, biscuits, chips, ice cream and other processed foods low in protein, micronutrients and fibre. But isn't it more helpful to say that these foods simply contain fewer nutrients than others? Despite being low in nutrients, they still give you energy and joy – which is the opposite of emptiness. Food is so much more than numbers and nutrients. It's also a source of comfort and satisfaction. Suppose you enjoy a food that isn't exceptionally nutritious or high in protein or modest in calories. In that case, if it fills your heart with joy, you can keep including it in your diet.

Involving calories in these discussions only serves to confuse. A calorie is and always will be a unit of measurement that measures the amount of energy you eat, irrespective of the food quality. The balance of calories in vs out over time defines your bodyweight. Micronutrients and fibre serve health by supporting your bodily functions, not your bodyweight. Energy and nutrients are both important, but their roles are independent of each other; they don't serve each other. The 200 calories in a doughnut are precisely the same as 200 calories in broccoli. It is the ratio of macronutrients and volume of micronutrients and fibre that make the two foods very different. I'll come back to this in the next section.

Food is so much more

than numbers

and nutrients.

WHAT ABOUT
MICRONUTRIENTS AND FIBRE?

Different foods contain varying levels of micronutrients, the vitamins and minerals essential for an array of critical bodily functions geared towards optimizing health and contributing to disease prevention. These are typically found in whole foods such as fruits, vegetables, legumes, meats, fish and dairy. An avocado, egg or chicken breast will contain more micronutrients than pastry, cookies or chocolate. Fibre is found in more whole foods than processed foods and is hugely important for gut health and can help you feel fuller. Fibre is typically found in carbohydrate-based foods like fruits, vegetables, bran, oats and beans. So, what does all this mean?

As we've seen, we burn more calories digesting high-protein foods than low-protein foods. But what if we compare 100g steak (high in protein) and 100g strawberries (low in protein)? The steak has 180 calories, and the strawberries only have 30. The protein in the steak means not all 180 calories will be absorbed. Nevertheless, the number of calories you will consume eating the steak will still be much, much higher than the 30 calories from the strawberries, regardless of the higher protein in the steak. The calories still count.

LOW-CALORIE
BARGAINS

Reducing calories doesn't necessarily mean you need to eat less. In fact, you can eat much more food than you did before and still create a calorie deficit. The key is understanding which foods are calorie-dense and which are calorie-sparse. For example, nuts, fatty meat, smoothies and nut butters contain a lot of calories in small amounts. Whereas fruit, vegetables, lean meat and fish contain fewer calories in large servings.

'NOT MUCH'	MUCH MORE

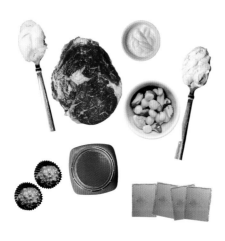

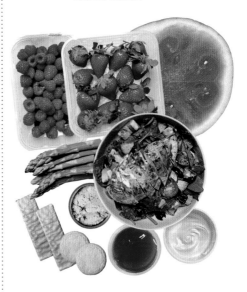

120g muffin, 50g mayonnaise, 50g brazil nuts, 50g macadamia nuts, 2 chocolates, 500ml fruit smoothie, 4 mini millionnaire's shortbreads (80g), 30g coconut oil & 30g peanut butter

200g chicken breast + mixed salad, 300g strawberries, 150g raspberries, 500g watermelon, 100g asparagus, 60g tuna, 400g low-calorie jelly, 200g 0% fat Greek yogurt, 2 ginger biscuits & 2 chocolate wafers

2,821 cal

972 cal

*Much **lower** volume of food, much **higher** volume of calories

*Much **higher** volume of food, much **lower** volume of calories

The simplest option

Do you have to count calories to lose weight? No. Does it make it easier? Yes, it makes you more informed. Given calories are made up of protein, carbs and fats, many people choose to track all three macronutrients instead. Though this is valid, it requires unnecessary diligence. The science says that we burn the highest number of calories eating protein, and that there's no difference in calories burned when eating low-fat or low-carb diets.[2] So isn't it easier, more logical and achievable to simply track calories and protein? You may ask, 'If tracking the calories that you consume is a good way to achieve fat loss, surely tracking the calories you burn is just as useful, right?' Here's why the answer to that is a resounding no.

It's enough effort to track the calories you consume, so trying to track calories you burn would double your workload. Additionally, attempting to track calories burned is pointless. When you get the calorie target from my website (www.fitnesschef.uk) it has already factored in how many calories you burn every day. Put simply, the calculator uses your age, sex, height, weight and activity level to work out roughly how many calories you burn each day from all movement, exercise, digesting food and simply existing. As the number of calories you burn each day will be the amount of calories you need to consume to maintain your weight, my calculator deducts 15 per cent from this figure to create a gradual calorie deficit. It's that simple. You don't need to do any funky maths on your own.

Attempting to track

calories burned

is pointless.

CALORIES OUT

So far, we've discussed in-depth one half of the simple energy balance equation – calories consumed – but what about the calories you expend? These are just as relevant and important to understand.

Total daily energy expenditure (TDEE) = the total amount of calories you burn every 24 hours.

TOTAL DAILY ENERGY EXPENDITURE (TDEE)

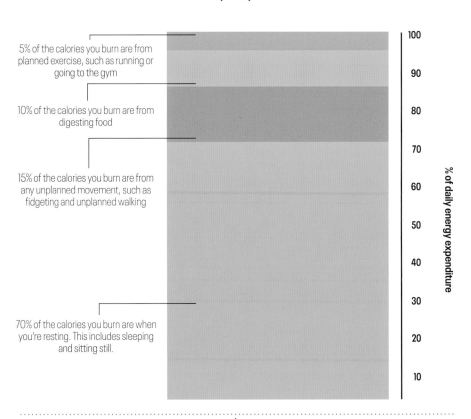

5% of the calories you burn are from planned exercise, such as running or going to the gym

10% of the calories you burn are from digesting food

15% of the calories you burn are from any unplanned movement, such as fidgeting and unplanned walking

70% of the calories you burn are when you're resting. This includes sleeping and sitting still.

% of daily energy expenditure

100
90
80
70
60
50
40
30
20
10

EATING AND EXERCISING
DON'T DEPEND
ON EACH OTHER

In 2020, I watched a programme showing how long you'd have to exercise to burn off certain meals. Presenters claimed that to burn off a 760-calorie meal you'd have to spend 95 minutes on a rowing machine. But given that we're constantly burning calories, even at rest, why would we need to pound exercise equipment for 1½ hours to cancel out the calories we've just eaten? I don't know about you, but I'd be content to burn off those 760 calories when I sleep – 8 hours should do it for me.

The psychological relationship between eating and exercise should never be co-dependent. This controlling behavioural trait is that of an eating disorder. Not only is the idea of earning calories from exercise hugely problematic, but it can lead to you believing you need to punish yourself for eating. We need calories to remain alive, yet, as shown opposite, we will continuously burn calories with or without exercise. Exercise exists to be enjoyed, not as a means to punish ourselves for overeating. If you don't exercise, you still need food as you're constantly burning calories. Make sure that any exercise you choose is something you enjoy first and foremost.

We will continuously

burn calories with

or without exercise.

Do I need an activity tracker?

Many calorie-tracking apps claim to be able to tell you that you're burning a specific number of calories each time you go for a run, walk or gym session. This is just an estimate. It's better than nothing, but not accurate according to a systematic review that found that the most popular activity trackers overestimated energy expenditure, with 50 per cent accuracy for jogging but much higher accuracy for walking. [3][4]

That said, activity trackers are still hugely beneficial as tools that increase our motivation to move more. This behaviour directly increases energy expenditure. Unlike calories consumed, not knowing the specific number of calories you're burning from exercise doesn't actually matter. There is not much value in trying to track every elusive calorie burned. It's more important to know your TDEE. Most daily calorie calculators already factor in estimated energy expenditure to the figure they give you. Yes, it's that simple. You don't need to subtract the calories your app tells you that you're burning from exercise from your overall calorie target – the calorie target is all you need to follow.

Don't worry about the detail, not least because it's going to be inaccurate anyway, even if it appears logical. Your motivation when exercising should be to become more flexible, build strength, achieve new personal bests and reduce the risk of developing conditions like osteoporosis as you age, not to burn calories or punish yourself. A recent systematic review concluded that exercise in all forms, whether it's walking or taking part in rigorous activity, has a beneficial effect on depressive symptoms in the general population across all ages.[5] This suggests that, aside from burning calories, exercise can be used as an important tool to benefit your mental health.

WHY PLANNED STRENUOUS EXERCISE IS UNLIKELY TO MAKE A BIG IMPACT ON YOUR WEIGHT LOSS

The fact is that around 70 per cent of the calories you burn every day are burned without you doing anything – because you are asleep, watching TV, driving or sitting at a desk. Just 5 per cent of our daily energy expenditure comes from planned, proactive exercise. This is because intense exercise is usually only sustainable for a short time. For example, high-intensity interval training (HIIT) can only last for 15–30 minutes or lifting weights for a few sets of reps that last a few seconds at a time.

Accounting for the second-largest percentage of your TDEE is non-exercise activity thermogenesis (NEAT). In short, this means anything from fidgeting, household chores or light walking. Given these movements aren't strenuous, they are relatively easy to increase and serve to burn a significant chunk of calories. Instead of dreading hardcore DVD workouts or beastly PT sessions, how about aiming to achieve 10,000 steps per day, which equates to roughly 1½–2 hours of walking. If you wear a step tracker, you'll be amazed how easy it is to rack up the steps going about your day-to-day life. Suppose you receive a 30-minute phone call every day. That's probably 30 minutes you could walk and talk, clocking up 1,500–2,000 steps with ease. Repeated a few times a week this equals a significant increase in energy expenditure with minimal effort. It's the opposite of psyching yourself up for the gym, but just as effective and arguably more sustainable. A study found that people with an active lifestyle could burn 2,000 calories more per day without planned exercise.[6]

DAILY ACTIVITY ENERGY EXPENDITURE

WORKING OUT

fidgeting, walking dog, ironing, washing, making food, house chores, pacing during phone calls

With planned exercise taking up only 5 per cent of your daily energy expenditure, is it that important? Yes and no. Yes, because although it's only a small fraction, it's likely to be intense and will burn a chunk of calories. No, because you can still burn many calories across the remaining 95 per cent of your energy expenditure. Increasing your protein intake and NEAT are just two simple ways to do this. Do you need the perfect training programme? No. You just need to show up.

Forget what you're told to do. What do you enjoy doing? If it's being outdoors, walking or climbing hills, those old clothes you have? They are just fine. The old trainers? Fine too. Buying expensive gym equipment because you think you need to do things perfectly is not a wise investment if you're not interested in them in the first place. Instead, use your body and the environment around you to create your own free workouts. There are no set rules as to what exercise or activity you should do to lose weight, but one rule you should definitely set yourself is to choose things you enjoy and that you can do regularly. Let's say you are female, 5ft 7in and weigh 80kg. By clocking up 10,000 steps every day you would burn approximately 350–450 calories alone. My guess is that this would be more than a gym-based workout.

If you enjoy gym environments, join a gym. But make sure you're comfortable with the equipment on offer and the people who frequent it so you look forward to turning up. Having a sense of community can spur you on. If you invest in a personal trainer, make sure they aren't milking money from you without delivering useful programmes, tips and advice. They should be providing you with the framework to one day train comfortably on your own. If you're still with the same PT after a year and you haven't progressed as you'd like, it's not working.

In recent years many have debated whether resistance training (weight training) or cardio is better for fat loss. The answer is simple, neither are better. Whether it's squats, bench press, jogging or high intensity interval training, the key is enjoying the activity enough to keep repeating it. That said, in my personal opinion, weight training has an advantage over cardio. As well as burning calories, it gives you the opportunity to progress varied, dynamic movements and overloads that make you stronger for day-to-day life. When you build muscle, you also burn more calories at rest. Don't underestimate the power exercise has on improvements in your mental health.

WHY AIMING
FOR IMPERFECTION WORKS

So-called perfect diets are likely to fail in the long term because perfection is a temporary phenomenon. It's also challenging to measure, and what is difficult to measure is ultimately difficult to achieve. You don't need to be perfect. Striving for perfection demands the utmost micro-focus on many different things at once, over and over and over again. As I'll discuss later, some of these demands might not even be relevant to weight loss at all. Changing your behaviours to achieve something new is a challenge. So, making the challenge too difficult too soon doesn't bode well for long-term success. When people argue that most diets fail, it's not because we are simply incapable of losing weight. It's because we select unsustainable dieting methods which fail to build supportive long-term habits over time. How many diets would fail if we undertook dietary changes that we understood and enjoyed? How successful and happy could we be if we were informed, realistic and self-caring? I suspect a lot more.

So-called 'perfect'
diets are likely to fail
in the long term.

Start at the beginning. Build the foundation of your dieting mindset by understanding that you must have a calorie deficit. It might help you to track the calories you eat, at least temporarily, so you can measure your adherence to the deficit. You don't need to turn your life upside down. You've already got a diet. To support it physically and mentally, you might just need to understand it a little better.

The equation is simple – getting there isn't as straightforward. Humans aren't perfect. Not because we are lazy, slack or poorly educated. The number of possible variables and influences on any decision you make can be endless. For anyone seeking the perfect diet, my question is: perfect for what? Optimal health? Improved energy? Decreased mortality? Increased life expectancy? Enjoyment? Convenience? Happiness? Supporting each of these things every time you eat is impossible. Remember, it's a game of averages. Your diet cannot give you all of these things at the same time. Your diet can't protect you against everything. You could eat nothing but whole foods for ten years and still get hit by a bus and die at the age of 35. Getting stressed about individual eating episodes is a waste of time. Individually, each one has about as much significance for your overall health as a grain of sand in the context of an entire beach.

This section can serve as the crucial first step to resetting your diet mindset and trusting yourself with the simple principles required to lose weight. We'll build on this in the following chapters. Now we're off the mark, it's time for the next step.

YOUR FAT-LOSS FOUNDATIONS

●

Calculate your calorie deficit
using a reliable online calculator.

●

Create a gradual decrease in calories consumed
by tracking calories and sticking to the target
the calculator gives you.

●

Increase your protein and fibre intake
to increase energy expenditure
and feel fuller for longer.

●

Implement small diet and lifestyle changes
that are easy to stick to.

●

Be flexible and relaxed in your mindset –
failure doesn't exist and there is always tomorrow
to help you stay on track.

●

Choose activities and exercise that you enjoy
and that you can sustain while increasing your daily step count.

●

Aim to be imperfect.
There's no need to put pressure on yourself.

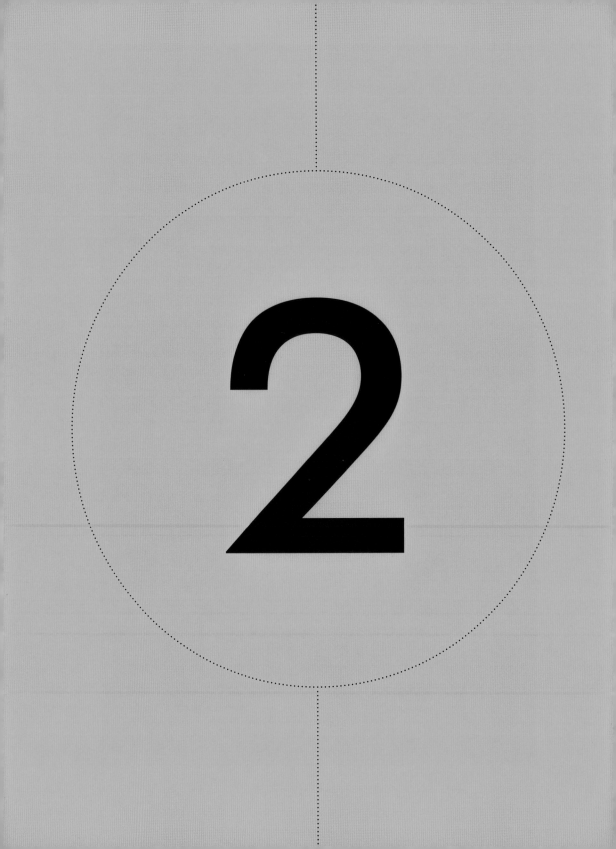

WHY THERE ARE NO 'GOOD' OR 'BAD' FOODS

BANNING FOODS:
THE VOLCANO EFFECT

'This food is good for you.'
'That food is bad for you.'

Whenever someone says this, challenge them. Ask them: why? If the food is not harmful or poisonous, how is it bad? Which specific ingredients are harmful? Is this dose going to harm you and what good or bad things will happen when you eat it? Hold them to coming up with answers to these simple questions. I guarantee they won't be able to.

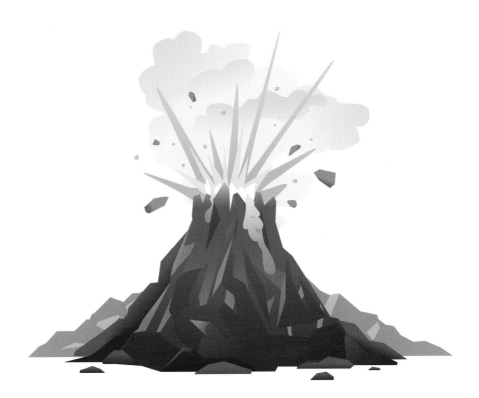

The fact that food is now commonly classified as good or bad for you reveals a fundamental problem in our diet culture. We are so focused on the health benefits of individual foods that we forget to consider the context. We rarely talk about food in context, yet it is context that determines how a food contributes to a person's health.

In the context of your life, individual eating episodes are insignificant. You won't gain fat by eating one doughnut or adding a spoonful of sugar to a drink, or even from consuming a 50g bag of sweets three times a week. Neither will that broccoli make you lean, and you can't rely on a cup of green tea each morning to improve your overall health.

Take Jen. She bases her new diet on whole, nutrient-rich foods. She also exercises most days and has a good sleep routine. Usually, Jen enjoys chocolate three times a week but to try to reach her weight-loss goal she decides not to eat it at all. Banning it from her diet means that she is omitting something she enjoys. Eventually, in a discouraged moment, Jen binges on a large quantity of chocolate, following which she feels consumed by guilt and shame.

But the chocolate didn't undo the healthful benefits of the whole foods she ate, or the quality sleep she had or the exercise she did. If Jen thought about chocolate in relation to her overall diet, instead of classifying it as a 'bad' food, she would understand that it is possible to enjoy chocolate with no adverse effects on her weight or overall health. Although the chocolate isn't as nutritious and filling as some foods, it doesn't necessarily mean Jen can't indulge in it as part of a nutritious and filling diet. It was her self-imposed chocolate ban that caused Jen problems.

If I tell you not to think of a bright yellow bear, what did you just do? You thought of a bright yellow bear. The instruction not to do something puts the idea into your head. The more Jen focused on not eating chocolate, the more she focused on chocolate – the less enjoyable her diet became, the more she thought about the food that brought her joy. This opened the door to a volcano effect whereby misery from restriction built up so much that she caved in and ate chocolate, and lots of it. If Jen spent less time desiring and thinking about chocolate and satisfied that desire in a way that supported her overall diet, it would reduce the chances of Jen's inner volcano erupting.

In Jen's case, ultra-restriction led to binge eating. Including chocolate regularly would have satisfied her desire for it and reduced the time she thought about it. She could have eaten it little and often and moved on with her day each time, benefiting her mental health and avoiding any potential for emotional turmoil, guilt-laden binges or shame. Research by food psychologists has referred to such eating binges and a preoccupation with food as an unanticipated consequence of self-imposed food restriction. Furthermore, that severe restriction appears to result in eating binges once food is available, resulting in psychological manifestations such as preoccupation with food and eating, increased emotional unease and distractibility.[8]

It is context that determines how a food contributes to your health.

ONE DOUGHNUT
WON'T RUIN YOUR SUMMER

Over time, Jen came to realize that eating chocolate (and by now I hope you know I mean any food) would not undo the healthful benefits of the more nutritious foods she ate. Rather than letting one food choice define her health, she saw it in the context of overall foods, nutrients, fibre, protein, sleep, stress, movement, exercise and mental health. There is simply no good evidence that suggests any single eating episode can negatively affect health. Dogmatic beliefs were useless to her but enjoying each food choice brought her calm and happiness.

If Jen is faced with friends, family or colleagues telling her she's bad for eating something, now she can confidently ask the accuser why. If the accuser reels off generalized claims, she knows she can safely ignore what is simply the referral of misinformation. Because she knows that there is no evidence to support that eating a single doughnut has any meaningful effect on overall health, good or bad. Instead, there is evidence that eating a diet rich in micronutrients, protein and fibre via a variety of nutritious animal produce low in saturated fat and plants does benefit overall health and help to reduce the risk of poor health. So, the good news is that the odd doughnut, or pastry, or any enjoyed, nutrient-sparse, processed, high-calorie food can be part of your diet, as long as the quantity of it you consume over time is moderate. One doughnut or one avocado won't mean you had a bad summer. What you ate over the entire summer is what counts.

WHAT YOU THINK

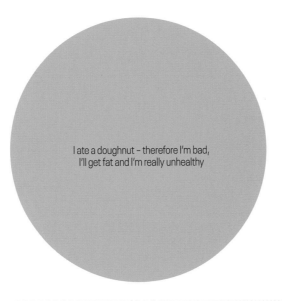

I ate a doughnut – therefore I'm bad,
I'll get fat and I'm really unhealthy

THE REALITY

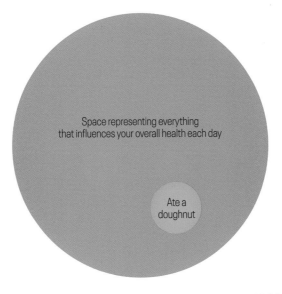

Space representing everything
that influences your overall health each day

Ate a
doughnut

WHY THERE ARE NO 'GOOD' OR 'BAD' FOODS

SUPER SIZE ME PROPAGANDA

In 2003, American Morgan Spurlock made a film about the health effects of eating three McDonald's meals a day for 30 days in a bid to investigate the US obesity epidemic. At the end of the experiment, Spurlock had gained weight, had increased cholesterol, reported mood swings and even sexual dysfunction.

So what were the findings of this experiment? Well, we found out that if you eat highly processed, calorie-dense food for every single meal, accept super-size portions when offered and live a sedentary lifestyle across 90 consecutive meals for 30 days, there's a good chance you'll gain body fat and your health markers will go down. But, given the extreme nature of this experiment, is this any surprise? Most, if not all, of us will not be consuming fast food three times a day, every day – so how useful is this experiment?

Suppose you enjoyed fast food once a week every month. That's four out of 90 meals per month comprising fast food compared to the 90 fast-food meals in this experiment. That's a huge difference. Unfortunately, this documentary led many to believe that eating McDonald's and other fast food causes obesity. It showcased the negative impacts that eating fast food for every single meal can have on your health, helping to spread a narrative that fast food is bad in any context. The more balanced truth is that if you are eating plenty of nutritious whole foods, you can still enjoy fast food occasionally if you want and maintain good health.

REMOVING MORALS
FROM FOOD
MAKES YOU SMARTER

Choice (noun) means the act of choosing between two or more possibilities, and if you're in a position to make your own food choices, you are privileged. In 2020, 720–811 million people on this planet faced malnourishment and hunger. In the same year, over 30 per cent of the world faced moderate or severe food insecurity.[9] The very fact that we can call a food healthy, unhealthy, good or bad, highlights the freedom and luxury we have to choose between different foods in the first place.

Despite the variety of tastes you've enjoyed over the years, social occasions built around feasts and comfort food from your favourite cookbooks, your relationship with food is simply that you need it to remain in existence. The sheer might of human cognitive development and the urge to explore has given us amazing flavours and textures to enjoy eating the world over. Well... some you will enjoy and some you won't. Let taste be your basis for classifying foods as good or bad and let go of food morality.

Your relationship with
food is simply that
you need it to remain
in existence.

THE 21 MEALS
OVER 7 DAYS FIX

Let's assume your goal is fat loss and eating a nutritious diet, and your fat-loss calorie target is 1,800 calories per day. Over a week you eat three main meals per day – that's 21 meals. For one of those meals, you are offered the choice between a 1,000-calorie pepperoni and cheese pizza or a 400-calorie chicken, lettuce, tomato and cucumber salad. Science tells us the pizza is calorie dense, less nutritious and contains 90g processed meat, despite guidelines suggesting you should consume no more than 70g per day to reduce your risk of colon cancer, and 35g saturated fat, despite recent guidelines saying you should aim to consume no more than 20g per day. The salad is relatively low in calories and a lot more nutritious as it contains a variety of vegetables, a lean source of protein and fibre. Which choice supports fat loss and overall health? The salad? That's a fair call. But what if I asked you which choice supports fat loss and overall health in the context of 21 meals spanning seven days? Still going with the salad? That's a fair call.

Shall I tell you my answers to both questions? OK, here goes. The salad is not a better choice than the pizza because in the context of 21 meals across seven days, the significance of the pizza is small. Yes, it means you likely exceeded your calorie target for one day, yes it exceeds processed meat and saturated fat guidelines in one eating episode. But once you invite context into the room you can understand that those 1,000 calories from the pizza are just 1,000 out of the 12,600 calories you can eat across seven days and still lose fat, just 90g processed meat out of 490g processed meat you can eat over the same period and avoid increasing your risk of colon cancer (according to the

> By applying science and context, you **can** eat your favourite calorie-dense meals.

WHY THERE ARE NO 'GOOD' OR 'BAD' FOODS

World Health Organization), and just 35g saturated fat out of the 140g recommended per week.

Rather than getting bogged down in unnecessary feelings of guilt or shame or believing that you have negatively affected your health (which may increase the likelihood of developing orthorexia, see page 81), you can shut them out by embracing the reality: you still have another 20 meals to achieve balance. If you only eat pepperoni and cheese pizza all week, that's a problem. If you only eat chicken salad all week, although it's slightly less of a problem, you're also missing out on many other important nutrients too (as well as probably being incredibly bored). By applying science and context, you *can* eat your favourite calorie-dense meals, knowing that you have the next meal as an opportunity to adapt and stay on track.

21 MEALS, 7 DAYS

Calorie target: 1,800 per day

MON	TUE	WED	THU

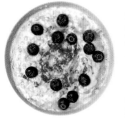 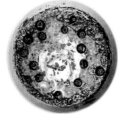 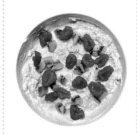 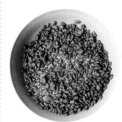

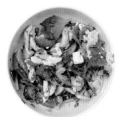 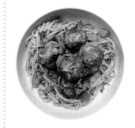 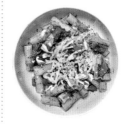 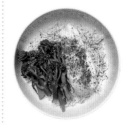

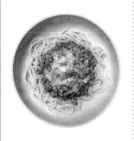 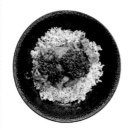 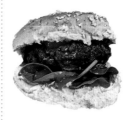 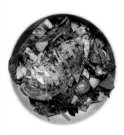

WHY THERE ARE NO 'GOOD' OR 'BAD' FOODS

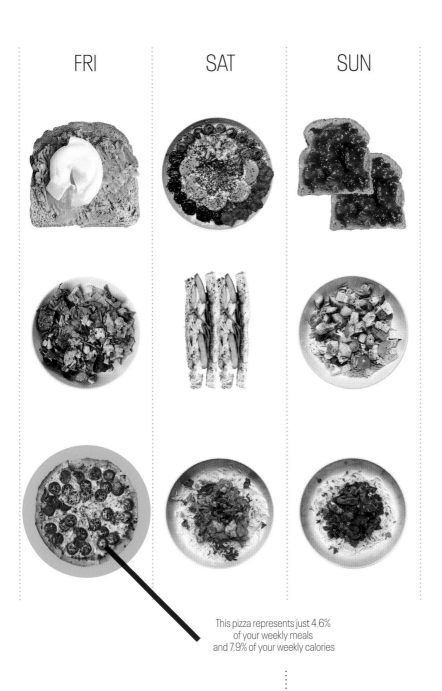

FRI	SAT	SUN

This pizza represents just 4.6%
of your weekly meals
and 7.9% of your weekly calories

WHY THERE ARE NO 'GOOD' OR 'BAD' FOODS

POISON IS IN THE DOSE,
NOT THE INGREDIENT

How many times have you heard someone call a particular ingredient or food 'toxic'? Or even poisonous? Perhaps they've told you not to eat it because it contains chemicals? Usually, these words are attributed to highly processed, low-nutrient foods and additives or preservatives that are hard to pronounce. It's very rare to hear someone say that a vegetable could kill you. Or that water can be fatal. A can of diet cola, however? That stuff is going to make your organs disintegrate, right? Many people believe it is poison in a can and that the chemicals it contains are dangerous. But can they tell us why? Can they name the poisonous chemicals or ingredients? Or the level of dose at which they become harmful to humans? Finally, can they cite any evidence to corroborate their claims?

It may surprise you to know that water contains chemicals and is also fatally poisonous. In other words, water can kill you. Alarming as it sounds that one of the essential things needed to sustain life could do the opposite; fortunately, this will only occur if you drink it in huge volumes. In 2007, in Los Angeles, Jennifer Strange tragically died hours after entering a water-drinking competition on local radio. The coroner concluded that she died of water intoxication, also known as hyponatremia. This can occur when the body's sodium levels drop low enough that water begins to dilute the sodium in the bloodstream, causing the brain to swell. In severe cases, it can result in coma or death. According to witnesses, Strange drank between 7 and 8 litres of water in just a couple of hours.

Too much of anything

can cause harm.

The point of this story is not to make you fear water, but to show that no matter how healthful the ingredient is, the danger is in the dose, not the ingredient. The same goes for those foods and drinks that don't offer abundantly beneficial properties. Too much of anything can cause harm, but if there's no evidence that harm exists in the consumed amount, how can these foods be harmful?

Poison or toxicity only occurs in a certain amount of the ingredient, not in the ingredient itself. For example, formaldehyde found in pears can be lethal, but not in the microscopic amount in a single pear, or even a dozen pears for that matter. Some people claim that food companies are loading their products with chemicals and toxins, poisoning you from the inside out. But it's funny how none of these people can name the alleged toxins or poisons, the dose at which they become toxic or poisonous, or the supposed harmful physiological results in your body. Without explicitly stating the above and backing it up with rigorous evidence, their claims are simply wild guesses and conspiracy theories.

YOU CAN'T
AVOID CHEMICALS

In June 2021, a British actress went on live TV to state that she went from a size 16 to a size 8 by doing the following:

- Counting chemicals, not calories.
- Removing vegetable and seed oils from her diet because they didn't allow her to digest other foods and triggered her depression, causing her to overeat.

Given this interview went out to an entire nation, it is important to pull this apart and put her words into context. Firstly, there is no science-based evidence that says any vegetable oils make us overweight or have any influence on how we metabolize other foods. Secondly, the actress

ARE 'CHEMICALZ' STILL BAD?

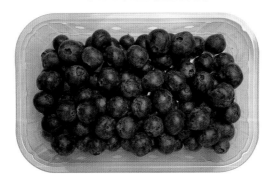

COMPOSITION OF BLUEBERRIES

Aqua, fructose, sucrose, fibre, E460, glutamic acid, aspartic acid, leucine, arginine, alanine, valine, glycine, proline, isoleucine, serine, threonine, phenylalanine, lysine, methionine, tyrosine, histidine, cystine, tryptophan, linoelic acid, linolenic acid, oleic acid, palmitic acid, stearic acid, plamitoleic acid, ash, phytosterols, oxalic acid, E300, E306, thiamin, E163a, E163b, E163e, E163f, E160a, ethyl ethanoate, 3-methyl butyraldehyde, 2-methyl butyraldehyde, pentanal, methylbutyrate, octene, hexanal, decanal, 3-carene, limonene, styrene, nonane, ethyl-3-methylbutanoate, non-1-ene, Texan-2-one, hydroxlinalool, lanalool, terpinyl, acetate, caryophyllene, alplha-terpineol, alpha-terpinene, 1,8-cineole, citral, benzaldehyde, methylparaben, 1510, E300, E400, E421, E941, E948, E290.

didn't seem to understand that chemicals and calories are completely unrelated. Calories are units of energy, while chemicals are compounds or substances. Even if chemicals were relevant to weight loss, how exactly do you count the chemicals in your daily diet? Counting calories isn't essential for weight loss, but it can be an incredibly useful tool. Counting chemicals for weight loss is not only entirely useless, but also nigh on impossible.

This 'chemical' fearmongering isn't limited to phony weight-loss advice. Many continue to argue that chemicals are making us unhealthy and in order to eat a healthful diet, there must be no chemicals present. The only problem is that everything on the planet contains chemicals – healthful and harmful. For example, water is made up of oxygen and hydrogen, chemicals we need to stay alive. Yes, diet cola and other artificially sweetened drinks contain chemicals, but just like the amount of oxygen or hydrogen in water, the quantity defines the safety. When claims arise that appear shocking or alarming, it's important to put them into context, and question them.

THE DETOX

Those who advocate juice cleanses, claiming they cleanse the body of toxins, fail to understand that as long as your liver, kidneys, lungs, gut and skin are functioning properly, they do this for you free of charge. In order to make their juicing detox plan relevant, those who promote them first have to convince you that you have a (fake) problem and that their juicing detox is the solution. It's unsurprising that many of these charlatans claim big food companies are poisoning you so you have to give money to Big Pharma to avoid ill health. It's all a conspiracy, right? Well, not quite. It sounds like a neat story, but it's merely a ploy to dismantle your trust in what you eat and how you're medically treated, which creates the illusion that juice cleanses are all of a sudden more appealing as a solution for weight loss and improved health. As long as you have working organs and a balanced diet, they really aren't – save your money and spend it on something worthwhile.

ARTIFICIAL INGREDIENTS

How many times have you heard either of these statements?

'Big food companies are out to get you with their fake food.'
'Eat real food, don't eat fake food.'

They might be born of good intentions, but the use of 'real' and 'fake' is pretty misleading. The latter statement may be followed with complaints about artificial flavours not being designed for human consumption, colours and additives that affect our brains, and preservatives that add toxins to our bodies. But while these things are not beneficial to our health, this doesn't mean that they harm it. Food free from colourings, additives and preservatives is abundantly more healthful and should be prioritized, but there is no evidence to suggest that these foods are toxic or harmful. The harm is always in the dose.

The word 'artificial' is the opposite of the word 'natural', so it is unsurprising that artificial ingredients are demonized by some of those consumed by the appeal-to-nature fallacy. This is essentially the argument that natural things are always good and unnatural things must always be bad. Many artificial flavours have the same chemical structure as naturally occurring flavours and enhance the taste of the food you eat. The word 'artificial' or 'unnatural' in and of itself says nothing about how safe a particular food is. By the same token, neither does 'real' or 'natural'. The box jellyfish is natural, yet lethal. A stinger suit is artificial, yet lifesaving.

The use of 'real'
and 'fake' is
pretty misleading.

If you can't pronounce it, you can still eat it

In mid-2021 I stumbled across a TikTok video where a 'health coach' was warning his nearly one million followers of the dangerous and harmful ingredients in baby formula made from cow's milk. He claimed the ingredients were dangerous and harmful because he couldn't pronounce them. However, upon closer inspection, a large quantity of the so-called harmful ingredients were simply chemical names for different proteins, carbs, vitamins and minerals that serve to benefit the nutritional needs of infants. The fact that you can or cannot pronounce an ingredient has no relevance to its safety.

INGREDIENTS IN BABY FORMULA

Organic Skimmed **Milk**, Organic **Whey** Product, Organic Vegetable Oils (Organic Palm Oil*, Organic Rapeseed Oil, Organic Sunflower Oil), Organic **Lactose**, Organic Galacto-Oligosaccharides from Organic **Lactose**, **Fish** Oil, Calcium Chloride, Potassium Citrate, Mortierella Alpina-Oil, Choline Sodium Citrate, L-Phenylalanine, Calcium Salts of Orthophosphoric Acid, L-Tryptophan, Magnesium Sulphate, Calcium Carbonate, L-Histidine, Zinc Sulphate, Ferrous Sulphate, Stabiliser Lactic Acid, Vitamin C, Vitamin E, Niach, Pantothenic Acid, Cuptic Sulphate, Vitamin A, Vitamin B1, Potassium Iodate, Vitamin B6, Folic Acid, Sodium Selenate, Vitamin K, Manganese Sulphate, Vitamin D, D-Biotin, Vitamin B12, *From sustainable organic production ·

mineral

adapted mineral for dental health

essential amino acid (protein)

vitamin B7

water soluble compound, similar to Vitamin B

mineral

plant sugars found in dairy, pulses and vegetables

used to prevent iron deficiency

used to prevent iron deficiency

also known as vitamin B5

essential amino acid (protein)

Food colourings

Colours used to change pigmentation in food are often heavily criticized. Scores of blogs claim that food colourings exacerbate attention deficit hyperactivity disorder (ADHD), particularly in children, warning parents of their hidden dangers. But a scientific meta-analysis found that only 8 per cent of children might have symptoms related to food colourings. Within this minority, it is still unclear if food colourings are the cause, rendering the link between ADHD in children and food colouring inconclusive.[10] Another study found that among children, adolescents and adults in the USA, the exposure to food colouring additives of both average and high-intake consumers was still well below the acceptable daily intake of each individual additive (as defined by the World Health Organization).[11]

In short: are food colourings healthful? No. Are they harmful? Not in the tiny doses present in the food that you or your child eats, although prioritizing whole, fresh food offers more benefits to overall health.

Preservatives

Preservatives don't inherently cause harm. In fact, salt is a preservative for meat and fish. In an ideal world, we would be given foods in their optimal states to eat before they spoil, but this isn't possible a lot of the time. It has been strongly argued that eating more than 70g cured or smoked meats and fish per day causes cancer. In 2015, The International Agency for Research on Cancer (IARC) classified them as group 1 carcinogens, alongside cigarettes, asbestos and arsenic. The IARC concluded that eating more than 50g cured, smoked or processed meat per day increased the risk of colon cancer by a whopping 18 per cent. However, a closer look at the IARC's classification system reveals that something resulting in a huge increased risk of cancer receives the same classification as something that increases risk by a tiny amount. As cancer scientist David Robert Grimes puts it in his book *The Irrational Ape:* 'the classifications do not convey how dangerous something might be, only certainty that it might be dangerous'. Looking closer at the data in the UK, 61 people per 1,000 develop colon cancer in their lifetime. For those who don't eat processed meat, the rate is 56 per 1,000.

WHY THERE ARE NO 'GOOD' OR 'BAD' FOODS

While for those who eat processed meat heavily, the figure is 66 per 1,000. Therefore, there are ten more colon cancers per 1,000 heavy processed-meat-eaters than 1,000 people who don't eat it at all. The IARC's figure of 18 per cent comes from determining the increased risk of heavy processed-meat-eaters relative to those who don't eat it at all. But given there were just 10 more colon cancers per 1,000 between the two groups, the absolute risk of eating lots of processed meat and getting colon cancer over the course of your lifetime is just 1 per cent. This doesn't mean eating unlimited quantities of smoked, cured or processed meat and fish is a good idea, but it may relieve some anxieties you have about eating it at all.

Some preservatives added to foods even help prevent foodborne illnesses, improving their safety. These are subject to extensive food safety tests. The idea that the senior figures of big food companies sit around a table and scheme ways to worsen our health is a baseless conspiracy theory. Furthermore, believing people are out to get you only increases your anxiety when making food choices. This is a slippery slope. You may have heard people claim that fast-food companies do extensive taste tests with the sole aim of making their food addictive. But could it be that they want their food to taste good, so more people enjoy it? Think of it like when you get ready for a date. You wouldn't spend all that time getting ready, only to purposefully not look your best and make a good impression. Instead, you may test different outfits until deciding on the one that you think you and your date will like best.

THE END OF IDOLIZING
AND DEMONIZING FOOD

When it comes to a single eating episode, the purpose is to provide energy for survival, pleasure for satisfaction and nutrients for wellbeing. Each food and the portions you eat them in may be different, but that's no reason to classify foods as good, bad, clean, dirty, healthy or unhealthy. These are not only unrelated moral descriptions, but they are also utterly useless to you. When you eat food, you (or it) cannot be morally good or bad. The only way food can be clean is to use cleaning products on it, which will actually make you seriously ill. The only possibility of food being dirty is if you drop it in mud or down the toilet. Being healthy or unhealthy is defined by your overall diet and other behaviours over months and years, not one meal. Words matter – they shape your beliefs. So, make sure you immerse yourself in calm, logical descriptions of the food you eat to find a balance of health, happiness and confidence.

Let's use the example of peanut butter on brown toast and strawberry jam on white toast. The peanut butter and brown bread are often idolized, and jam and white bread frequently demonized. Peanut butter offers many more nutrients and satiating qualities than the jam, and brown bread contains more fibre than white bread. But it's one choice out of many hourly, daily, weekly, yearly choices made over decades – the significance of this single choice on your health at one point in time is virtually zero.

You cannot swim to new

horizons until you have

courage to lose sight of

the shore. WILLIAM FAULKNER

BEING 'GOOD'

BEING 'BAD'

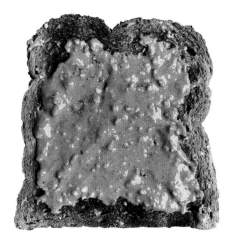

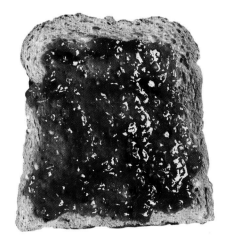

40g peanut butter
on 40g brown toast

**40g strawberry jam
on 40g white toast**

334 cal

194 cal

*Viewing the food you eat in the context of enjoyment, energy and nutrients across your overall diet
allows you to realize that there are no good or bad foods – only different foods offering different things

In this example, 40g peanut butter on a slice of brown bread (a typical portion size) works out at 334 calories; 40g strawberry jam spread on a slice of white bread (another common portion) works out at 194 calories. The peanut butter on toast may be a good idea if you aim to consume more nutrients and feel fuller, but the jam spread on toast can support a calorie deficit better as it contains fewer calories. Or, if you want to eat the peanut butter and eat something nutritious, reducing the amount would better help to create a calorie deficit.

When a rival sports team scores a fantastic goal against your team, the other supporters celebrate while you sit in despair. But the neutral supporter appreciates the goal for its brilliance and relevance in the context of the match. Your food beliefs should be no different. Don't get bogged down in individual eating choices. You need to think about them within the context of your overall diet. If you get too caught up in the small stuff, you lose sight of the big picture.

//

If you get too caught up in the small stuff, you lose sight of the big picture.

//

FOOD QUALITY MATTERS
FOR OVERALL HEALTH

One day, you're going to die. I know, I said it, but it's the truth. If anything, this fact should help you to ensure you make the most of the time you have. You can eat any food you desire throughout your life, no matter what it is. If certain foods please you, then eat them solely for that reason. That said, to optimize your health and live a long, healthful life, there are some considerations to bear in mind.

THE MEANING OF MICRONUTRIENTS

Micronutrients, aka vitamins and minerals, are essential for your wellbeing. Even chocolate contains some micronutrients, but nowhere near enough for overall health if it's your only micronutrient source. Foods like fruit, vegetables, legumes, beans, nuts, dairy, meat and fish contain much higher volumes of many different micronutrients that benefit your health and help prevent disease. In a critical review of the effect fruit and vegetables have on preventing chronic disease, the researchers concluded that there was convincing evidence that high daily intakes of fruit and vegetables reduce the risk of developing hypertension, cardiovascular disease and strokes. The review concluded that there was probably evidence that high daily intakes also reduce the risk of cancer.[12] It's worth saying that the onset of these diseases and conditions depend on multifaceted genetic, dietary and lifestyle behaviours over long periods, but getting an adequate intake of fruit and vegetables and other nutrient-dense foods seems like an easy way to reduce this risk. It is widely agreed that you should aim to eat 7–10 portions of fruit and vegetables per day; 80g represents a portion of each, though exceeding this is not a problem.

A meta-analysis also showed that increasing intake of fruit and vegetables promoted weight-loss and prevented weight gain in overweight or obese individuals.[13] This is no doubt down to the fact that replacing high-calorie foods with those lower in calories helps to create a calorie deficit over time. The next time someone tells you that eating fruit is bad, kindly present them with these heavily researched findings.

FIBRE IS YOUR FRIEND

The other upside to eating fruit, vegetables and other carb-based whole foods is fibre. Not only is a high fibre intake shown to reduce your risk of colon cancer, but digesting it is also important in maintaining a healthy gut. A systematic review found that there is growing evidence to suggest that 47 per cent of colon cancer cases could be prevented with a more healthful lifestyle, and risk of colon cancer could be reduced by up to 20 per cent if adequate fibre is consumed.[14] It is widely recommended that you aim to eat 25–30g fibre per day. Fibre is typically dense in foods like fruit, vegetables, beans, pulses, unrefined grains, oats, nuts, potatoes and cereals. Foods high in fibre are also harder for your body to digest, meaning that you burn more calories digesting them, and they tend to make you feel fuller too. This reduces the likelihood of overeating and can help support your calorie deficit for weight loss.

A NOTE ON THE GLYCAEMIC INDEX (GI)

Many have been led to believe that following a low glycaemic diet can support weight loss and overall health. But let's take a look at what it is and put it into context. The glycaemic index (GI) rates foods containing carbs depending on their effect on your blood sugar after eating them. Foods high on this index include sugar, sugary drinks, potatoes and white rice. Foods lower on the scale are fruit, vegetables, pulses, beans and oats. It is often claimed that foods with a higher GI don't fill us up. While this is true when it comes to sugar, it isn't when it comes to potatoes. A study measuring satiety in common foods found that boiled potatoes ranked the highest out of grains, meat, fish, sweets and dairy products.[15] Though white rice may not be filling, what about if you ate it with a variety of vegetables and a source of protein? Nutritious, low-calorie watermelon is high on the glycaemic index, but less nutritious, calorie-dense fries and pastries are lower because their fat content slows down the body's absorption of carbs. If you're diabetic, following a low-GI diet may be beneficial as it can help to control blood glucose, otherwise, the question to ask yourself is whether the glycaemic index is useful for making food choices that support your weight and health goals.

FILLING FOOD

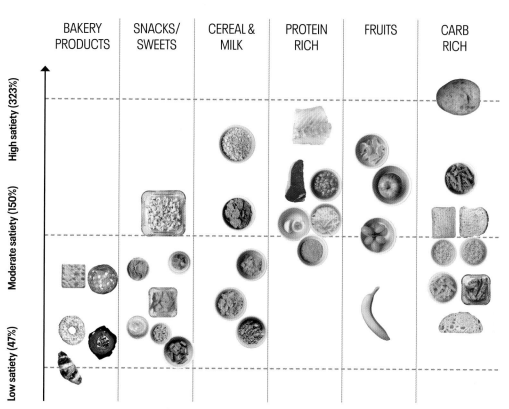

* Source study: 'A satiety index of common foods'

WHY THERE ARE NO 'GOOD' OR 'BAD' FOODS

POWERFUL PROTEIN

We've touched on the importance of protein earlier (see page 36); a macronutrient made up of amino acids that repairs tissues throughout the body. Eating 1–2g protein per kg of bodyweight each day supports your immune system and provides a constant drip-feed of important vitamins like B12, which plays an essential role in producing red blood cells. Vitamin B12 is usually found in animal products, which means that those following a plant-only diet may require B12 supplementation if deficient.

Consuming sufficient protein will also help you retain muscle mass, meaning you'll burn more calories at rest. Protein burns significantly more calories during digestion than carbs and fats (see page 34), increasing your energy expenditure to help fat loss. Lastly, protein tends to make you feel fuller, like fibre, improving appetite control and even aspects of mood and cognition.[16] Over and over, the body of evidence supports the consensus that diets higher in protein are associated with better health and lower body fat. A systematic review of 20 randomized control trials found that older adults retained more muscle and lost more fat when consuming higher-protein diets in conjunction with a calorie deficit.[17] If you feel hungry or sluggish maintaining your calorie deficit, consider increasing the amount of protein you eat each day by around 30 per cent, while keeping your calorie deficit the same. For example, if you are eating 70g protein every day, try increasing this to 90g to see if this reduces hunger and fatigue.

Diets high in protein are

associated with better

health and lower body fat.

HEALTHFUL
BARGAINS

Most whole, unprocessed foods offer multiple health benefits. Protein and fibre are entwined with physiological and behavioural aspects of weight control, too. Still, within this vast array of nutritious food, it's important to understand differences instead of believing that eating them in any quantity is a good idea. For example, most vegetables are low in calories and offer fibre and micronutrients. Beans are a moderate source of calories and protein and offer fibre and micronutrients. Chicken breast is a relatively low-calorie food, but also provides high amounts of protein and micronutrients. Avocado, oily fish and nuts are relatively high in calories, but a rich source of micronutrients. Understanding these differences will help you make supportive decisions for weight loss, good health and happiness over time.

MAKING ROOM
FOR NUTRIENTS

There's no evidence that processed foods like fast food, chocolate, sweets and refined carbs inherently cause disease or make you fat. So why do dietitians, doctors and mainstream media keep saying that they do? The answer is simple. These highly processed foods don't provide the same nutritional benefits that whole foods do. But just because something isn't beneficial doesn't mean it is automatically harmful. A recent systematic review found an association between the consumption of ultra-processed foods and the risk of disease onset.[18] But this doesn't mean eating ultra-processed foods in any capacity causes disease.

Consider this in context. A diet high in ultra-processed, low-quality food is simply less likely to allow space for enough nutritious foods that help us feel full and contribute to preventing ill health. It's not the chocolate, the pizza or the fries that cause disease or make you fat; it's the fact that eating more of these types of foods leaves less room for nutritious fruits, vegetables, pulses, beans, lean meat and oily fish that may help prevent the onset of disease, have satiating qualities and, over time, increase your energy expenditure to help control your weight.

Your average intake of nutrients and fibre, along with other aspects of your lifestyle, such as sleep and stress, can influence your overall health. One day of eating nutritious, high-quality food won't undo the effects of 30 days of non-stop consumption of ultra-processed, low-quality food, and vice versa. You want to find a balance for your physical and mental health.

A simple but effective strategy for maintaining a steady trickle of nutrients can come from two things you use almost every second: your memory and foresight. For example, suppose you eat a nutritious breakfast and lunch; you can enjoy a less-nutritious dinner if you like. If you ate a nutrient-poor breakfast, you could eat a nutritious lunch and dinner. If you eat a nutritious breakfast, lunch and dinner, you can then enjoy less nutritious snacks, if you like. Suppose you already know what you're going to eat for dinner. In that case, you can choose your meals earlier in the day to balance the quality and your enjoyment of the food you eat.

The key is understanding that a controlled intake of less-nutritious, processed food won't cancel out the nutrient-dense foods' benefits. If they still fit within your calorie target, they can be slotted in with ease, adding further enjoyment to your diet. No harm done.

Eating nutritious foods won't automatically make you lose weight unless you're in a calorie deficit. But if basing your diet on them means you feel full, burn more calories digesting them and feel less compelled to eat more than you need, then increasing whole foods could support your weight-loss goal. If you're informed about your food choices, it enables you to understand how they relate to your overall health, bodyweight and happiness.

IF THIS IS BEING
EXTREME

**THEN THIS IS ALSO BEING
EXTREME**

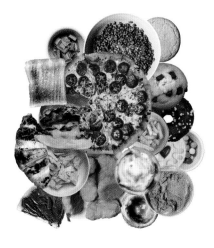 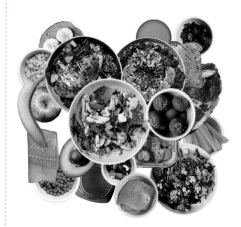

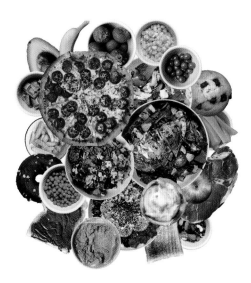

Prioritize nutritious whole foods because they will benefit your **overall
health**, but realize that just because processed foods often don't offer the
same benefits, it **doesn't** automatically make them harmful. You still have
unconditional permission to eat **ANY food** you **enjoy** to benefit your
mental health.

WHY THERE ARE NO 'GOOD' OR 'BAD' FOODS

THE
TAKE-HOMES

When people criticize your food choices or you are confronted by material that suggests certain foods are harmful, remember what we've covered in this section. Instead of succumbing to emotive jargon, critical thinking allows you understand that context and evidence govern the validity of your food choices. This liberates you to enjoy eating any food you wish, at any time you please.

It is impossible for food to be good or bad. Each food is simply different. Some have more calories; others have less. Some have more nutrients, others less. Some fill us up; others don't. Ultimately, the frequency and volume of food you eat will influence your physical and mental health. Don't let people insert baseless fearmongering into your food choices. At the very least, question someone on exactly why they claim a food is harmful. If they don't have a scientific, rational explanation, ignore them.

No food makes you gain fat or lose fat. The amount of body fat you have answers only to the number of calories you eat and burn. Severely restricting or banning foods entirely is more likely to lead to binge-eating behaviours and eventually excessive eating, not to mention feelings of deprivation, misery, guilt and shame. Your mental health is more than likely to take a massive hit.

No food inherently causes harm or disease, but too much of it might. Just as no food inherently benefits your health unless you eat enough of it. Aiming to eat 7–10 portions of fruit and vegetables alongside 25–30g fibre per day will leave more than enough scope to enjoy less nutritious foods in moderation. One salad's contribution to optimizing your health means far less if the other 20 meals consumed across the week are ultra- processed and low quality. Just like one takeaway's contribution to poor health means far less if the other 20 meals consumed that week were nutrient-rich and of high quality. You need to find a happy balance.

Don't let people insert
baseless fearmongering
into your food choices.

Unfortunately, many people in positions of authority, including those with large social-media followings, continue to argue that food can be good or bad, regardless of volume, frequency and quantities of specific ingredients. While it is important to promote the benefits of whole foods, it is not a free pass to demonize others. Perpetuating the idea that food has moral value only ends up with more and more people developing orthorexia, an eating disorder where you become obsessed with overeating nutritious foods, believing certain foods will cause harm.

These ideas fail or refuse to recognize context or evidence regarding the effects of eating different foods over time. Being accurately informed often depends on your ability to distinguish science from pseudoscience, truth from falsehood and logic from conspiracy. This is something we'll build on in the next section.

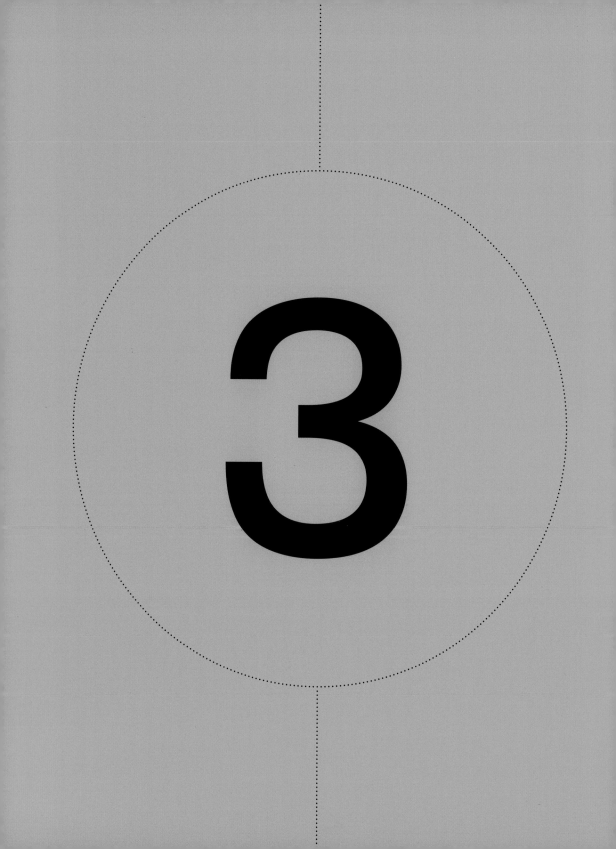

HOW
TO DROWN OUT
DIET
MISINFORMATION

PART 1

FINDING THE WHOLE TRUTH

CONFIRMATION BIAS

Confirmation bias is when you look for information that reinforces what you already think. Sally is in the habit of drinking 3–4 glasses of wine a night. She sometimes sees news stories about studies claiming a glass of wine is good for you, and she enjoys reading these. Although there are far more news stories about studies showing drinking several glasses of wine every day is not good for you, she doesn't notice these. The reports that say drinking a glass of wine is beneficial to health catch her attention because they confirm that her existing life choices are right.

I often see confirmation bias rear its head in the comments on my Instagram posts. Let's take fast food as an example. Too much fast food and not enough nutritious food can increase disease and obesity risk over time as fast food is low in nutrients and high in calories. This gets misinterpreted as any amount of fast food causes disease and obesity, so when angry_man69 (a private account, of course) sees a post reassuring people they can still eat fast food and have a healthful diet, he is outraged because it challenges his entrenched beliefs. His confirmation bias doesn't see any context and he's in no mood for critical thinking. If you politely mention there is no evidence that fast food causes disease or obesity, he won't hear you. His confirmation bias blinds him to a scenario in which somebody who eats sufficient nutrients and controls their calories can enjoy a small amount of fast food and still lead a healthful life. In fact, including it may improve diet enjoyment, thereby nourishing mental health.

So why do people form these beliefs? To understand this, we need to address the sources from which people form them.

Confimation bias is when you look for information that reinforces what you already think.

MEDIA
HEADLINES

Headline:
A glass of red wine every day can help prevent heart disease.

This is mainly down to research showing that resveratrol, a polyphenol known to help prevent heart disease, is present in red wine. The clickbait tabloid headline reads: 'Red wine prevents heart disease'. The natural reaction from those who drink regularly is pleasant surprise. This means we should all drink more red wine to improve our health, right?

Not so fast. The amount of resveratrol needed to make a meaningful difference in protecting you against heart disease would require you to drink so much red wine that you are more likely to suffer from alcohol poisoning before reaping any cardiovascular benefits. A study that looked into this found it's impossible to absorb the doses of resveratrol needed to have beneficial effects by drinking red wine.[19] But despite this being clearly stated in research, media headlines promoting red wine as a healthy drink continue, each one ignoring this crucial caveat. 'Drink red wine to avoid heart disease' is a sure-fire way to grab a reader's attention, sell more papers or get more views. While the media report a lot of accurate information, it's not all in the headlines.

> While the media report a lot of accurate information, it's not all in the headlines.

In June 2021, I noticed several newspapers reporting what they called a 'ground-breaking' new approach to kick-start obese people on their weight-loss journey. Researchers from the University of Otago in New Zealand invented jaw-locking clamps with custom-made bolts, allowing wearers to only open their mouths wide enough to drink liquids and so reduce their calorie consumption. As well as unethical and intrusive, many rightly pointed out that the device may cause you to choke to death in the event of vomiting. Resorting to this solution to lose weight is like applying a plaster to a widening crack, hoping it'll fix it. While those who sell the 'ground-breaking' plasters make money, you're left to deal with the ever-widening crack. Perhaps the journalists and editors didn't personally believe the device to be ethical or practical, but they needed eye-catching headlines to boost engagement.

This conflict of interest stretches far beyond red wine and jaw clamps. One day, there is a newspaper lauding fruit as a fat-burning food, only for the same newspaper to claim a few weeks later that fruit makes you fat. Another paper will say sugar makes you fat, the next week it's bread, then it's artificial sweeteners. They claim meat makes you fat and causes cancer, too. Even protein has been accused of being fattening, as bad as smoking and damaging to your kidneys. Each of these bold headlines doesn't tell the whole story of the science they are referring to. But these headlines devoid of context are leapt on as credible sources by those with hard-held beliefs as confirmation that they were right all along. Sugar must make you fat. Artificial sweeteners do kill you. Bread is bad. And the messages in these headlines speak to all of us – these are foods eaten regularly by everyone. With each repetition, we become more inclined to believe them.

As we've established, no food is harmful in itself. Yet, repeated exposure to misleading headlines could lead somebody who is otherwise eating a varied and healthful diet, enjoying sugar, bread and meat, to believe that they should abstain from eating them, damaging their relationship with food.

DOES THE EVIDENCE
STACK UP?

I came across Bayesian theory in a TED Talk by Alex Edmans, a Professor of Finance. It asks if the data supports the theory. For example, does rigorous scientific evidence underpin the theory that eating bread regularly makes you fat? It suggests that we tend to restrict our thinking to the theory being proposed. For example, we might conclude that because someone consumes bread regularly and is overweight, it must mean bread is the direct cause of their weight gain. Case closed?

No, the case is very much open. We have to consider 'rival theories'. What about people who also eat bread regularly who are not overweight? Due to confirmation bias, we typically fail to consider rival theories and the bigger picture because we want to protect our beliefs. We prefer embracing a single story to sifting through tons of data and we gravitate towards views that seem easier to believe and are more relatable.

In Professor Edmans' words, 'a single story is meaningless and misleading unless large-scale data backs it up'. No large-scale data supports the theory that eating bread makes you overweight. Not least because the quantity of bread has not even been considered yet. Is it one slice amounting to 100 calories every day for five years? Or is it ten slices amounting to 1,000 calories every day for five years? Both examples represent bread eating, but the calories consumed in both scenarios are massively different; 1,642,500 calories different, to be precise. This critical thinking allows us to see that excess calories cause fat gain, not bread.

TIPS ON EVALUATING EVIDENCE
TO MAKE UP YOUR OWN MIND

WHO IS IT BY?

The source of the research is usually cited in a reputable news piece, so you can check it out. Knowing this will help you find out if there is an agenda. For example, is the author a practitioner recommending you avoid all dairy to lose weight and who is also selling a dairy-free cookbook?

IS THE EVIDENCE SOURCE WIDELY AVAILABLE, PUBLISHED AND PEER-REVIEWED BY EXPERTS ON THE SUBJECT?

Is it just one source? Or is the evidence about the benefits of cutting out dairy for weight loss endorsed by many other experts from different nutritional and medical circles in many research papers?

KNOW THE DIFFERENCE BETWEEN CORRELATION AND CAUSATION.

An example of this can be found in articles claiming that eating red meat causes cancer. When looking closer at some of the evidence used to build this theory, you can see that red meat was eaten more by subjects who also smoked, which increases cancer risk. This means that red meat is correlated with cancer risk, but only because it was included in the same research. The idea that red meat, a food consumed globally, causes cancer is dynamite for media outlets to sell headlines to shock us. This headline is latched on to because it's easy to understand, and cancer is a highly emotive subject that many fear. Even if it lacks context, using scientific research is enough for many of us to believe a claim is credible. We tend only to share what sounds good (or, in this case, bad), regardless of the whole picture.

Think about this example for a second: arguing that correlation proves causation is the same as claiming that fire engines cause fires because they are always present when there's a fire. Critical thinking allows us to realize that fire engines don't cause fires; they do the opposite by putting them out.

THE CHECKLIST OF TRUTH

☐

If it's a story, is it true?

☐

If it's true, is it backed up by large-scale evidence?

☐

If it is, who is the research by?

☐

If you get two conflicting opinions from two different sources,
are you willing to embrace both equally rather than choosing
the one you want to be true?

Sometimes finding the truth is difficult. A lot of science is work in progress and filled with nuance. But to get the most reasonable, logical and tested answers, you need to put aside your ego and replace it with a willingness to sometimes be wrong. Respecting debates on both sides and finding the middle ground is vital to get the most accurate possible answer to a question. Usually, the most valuable scientific findings are the least extreme and suggest further research is required. The least valuable research is that which has not been tested much and has little evidence for the claims made.

Finding the middle ground is vital to get the most accurate possible answer.

Here is a brief guide to the best types of evidence sources available, free from bias or media sensationalism.

The hierarchy of evidence

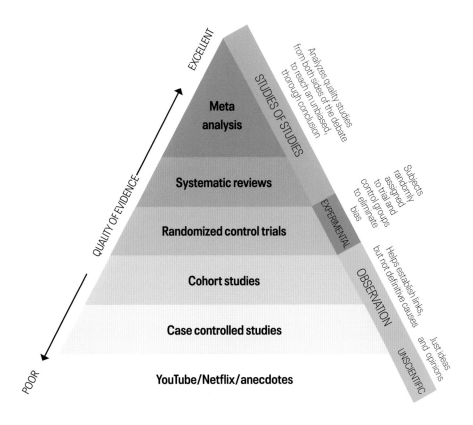

EXCELLENT

QUALITY OF EVIDENCE

POOR

STUDIES OF STUDIES

Meta analysis

Systematic reviews

Randomized control trials

Cohort studies

Case controlled studies

YouTube/Netflix/anecdotes

Analyzes quality studies from both sides of the debate to reach an unbiased, thorough conclusion

Subjects randomly assigned to trial and control groups to eliminate bias

EXPERIMENTAL

OBSERVATION

Helps establish links, but not definitive causes

UNSCIENTIFIC

Just ideas and opinions

WHY A WILLINGNESS
TO BE WRONG
CAN MAKE YOU SMARTER

Most animals are simple beings. They spend the majority of their lives eating, sleeping, sourcing food and shelter, raising their young and staying alert to danger. As humans, we are no different in these regards, but given our intellectual advancement, our sense of danger stretches beyond life and death. Our instincts may help protect us, but it is our beliefs that define who we are. If we believe something to be true, only to be told by someone that it isn't, we are hard-wired to defend our belief, no matter what it is. How helpful are these reactions? Sure, we may protect our egos, but closing doors and finding weak reasons for the sake of not being wrong about something comes at the cost of hindering our ability to acquire potentially helpful information.

Everything you've ever learned was the result of not knowing it in the first place. For example, like me, I'm assuming you believed there was a tooth fairy at one point in time. But as you got older, evidence and logic played out to make you change your mind. Perhaps you gathered more proof in the form of waiting up, only to witness your parents putting money under your pillow, or that fairies carrying endless coins didn't exist, let alone fly through the sky at night.

Today, you know how to read and write, but at one point, you didn't. You learned that skill when you went to school. The information we are exposed to, along with evidence, forms our beliefs. Sometimes we trust the information, no matter where it comes from, without consulting the evidence to validate it. We need to be willing to embrace the fact that sometimes we looked in the wrong place, causing us to be at least partially wrong about what we believed to be true at any one time. Perhaps a good anecdotal example of this is how you feel about a past relationship years after a break-up. At the time you thought you couldn't live without them. Years later you are thankful you did.

THE BURDEN OF PROOF

On one of my Instagram posts describing the calorie difference between Greek yogurt and 0 per cent fat Greek yogurt, someone commented: 'Stop promoting dairy; it's a carcinogen and causes cancer. Also, stop it already with promoting low-fat products that are full of chemical-laden ingredients that put you in hospital…'

I promptly replied, asking for the specific ingredients and chemicals he was referring to, along with the doses at which they became harmful and what harm occurs. After all, if it's so detrimental, this information should be readily available to share and help us all? I also pointed out that the only carcinogenic element in dairy is oestrogen, a hormone we produce naturally and in much higher doses than we will ever consume through dairy. I received a scathing retort, but my questions remained unanswered, with no evidence supporting his original claims. The burden of proof was on him, and his claims were meaningless without evidence.

The burden of proof refers to a scientific standard that requires anyone or any party to demonstrate that a claim is valid or invalid based on quality evidence. If someone claims that aspartame, an artificial sweetener used in zero-calorie drinks, causes cancer, metabolic disease or obesity, they need to provide compelling evidence to support this claim. Anything short of this is simply a theory, hypothesis or opinion, all of which are not solid proof.

Let's use sugar-free, artificially sweetened drinks as an example. The list of adverse side-effects purported by factions of the media, medical professionals, dietitians, scientists, researchers and the general public is long. Cancer, diabetes and obesity are three things reported to occur if you consume aspartame. But how accurate are these statements?

Well, in each of the cases above, not very. Despite recent observational research showing that artificial sweeteners are among the most talked about aspects of nutrition, a systematic review published in 2019 analyzing the negative health impact of artificial sweeteners concluded that there was insufficient evidence to associate them with a risk of cancer, diabetes or obesity.[20] While there was no compelling evidence to suggest that artificial sweeteners offered any health benefits, the fact they contain next-to-no calories and provide a sweet taste suggests that they could be an alternative for someone who enjoys regular soda, but wants to reduce body fat. The research that many on the other side of the argument seem to cling to was conducted on rodents. Possible links to blood cancers were found when rats were given several hundred times the aspartame contained in a single can of drink. But we are humans and unlikely to drink hundreds of cans of diet cola every day.

The only science that could be manipulated to support the idea that artificial sweeteners make us fat is correlating the artificial sweetener consumption of those who are overweight with their weight, without assessing other possible reasons why they are overweight. Fortunately, a second systematic review in 2020 and meta-analysis concluded that there were no bodyweight differences between those consuming low-calorie artificial sweeteners compared with those consuming zero-calorie water.[21]

Another claim in this debate is that sugar-free sweeteners trick your brain into thinking it has ingested sugar, thus raising insulin levels, leading to fat storage. This is simply impossible. Insulin is a hormone released by the pancreas to regulate blood glucose levels when calories are consumed. Given these sugar-free drinks don't contain calories, there is no meaningful insulin response. This falsehood stems from what's known as cephalic insulin response – our reaction to food cues. Some argue that because sugar and zero-calorie artificial sweeteners are both sweet, the brain detonates the same insulin response to both. A systematic review of cephalic phase responses to food cues found these responses biologically meaningless to everyday life.[22]

It's important to be aware that evidence is ever-evolving.

A fourth systematic review and meta-analysis published in 2020 concluded that aspartame was actually associated with fat loss and didn't negatively affect blood sugar or insulin compared to those who drank water instead.[23]

This isn't to say aspartame-sweetened drinks are better for your health than water, but the data clearly shows that they don't cause the harm that many claim they do.

Lastly, many have claimed that artificial sweeteners negatively affect gut health. But a randomized control trial suggested that typically high consumption of aspartame and sucralose, the two most commonly used sweeteners, had minimal effect on gut microbiota in humans. More research is required.[24]

The multitude of high-quality evidence above clearly shows that unless you drink hundreds of cans of fizzy drinks a day, drinking artificially sweetened drinks containing aspartame, or other sweeteners will not harm your health unless you're allergic to them. Will they benefit your health? Not necessarily. But given that they contain next-to-no calories, they could help you lose weight if you previously drank a higher-calorie version.

Case closed? Well, not quite. While the highest-quality evidence is always the best route to being well informed, it's important to be aware that evidence is ever-evolving. At some point, future research on aspartame may tell a different story. But using this as a reason not to trust the current evidence would be like saying pigs fly today because one day they might. We'll have to wait and see how that one pans out, but for now, the burden of proof lies with those who claim artificial sweeteners cause cancer, diabetes and obesity, despite the body of evidence suggesting otherwise.

BE PREPARED TO WEATHER
THE STORM OF HALF-TRUTHS

Imagine you're in a café with your friend and you order your favourite milkshake. Your friend turns to you and says, 'I wouldn't drink that if I were you, I heard dairy causes inflammation, which can lead to cancer and loads of health issues.' You'd be at least a little disconcerted, right? At worst, you'd think that this one milkshake may cause you serious health issues. At best, you might think you should make this the last time you enjoy your favourite milkshake before you completely cut out dairy.

Before the milkshake apocalypse begins, consider this. In a large-scale clinical review of dairy products and inflammation, it was found that dairy doesn't cause inflammation at all. It concluded that dairy is anti-inflammatory,[25] even for those suffering from metabolic disorders.[26] So, how did this complete 180-degree falsehood come about? There is some evidence suggesting that dairy can be inflammatory for those who are allergic to it. But the same goes for any food we are allergic to, not just dairy.

This is an example of advice purported as healthful, potentially turning out to be harmful if we aren't careful. As well as being anti-inflammatory, dairy is rich in protein and a host of other essential micronutrients such as B12 and calcium that are important for overall health, albeit from more nutritious sources than a milkshake.

OPEN YOUR EYES

Last year I did an Instagram post showing four nutritious snacks: a flapjack; a nut-based snack bar; 60g Brazil nuts and 250ml fruit smoothie. Though challenging to picture, I can assure you that it's not much food. I reported that the four snacks totalled 1,231 calories and mentioned they contained a lot of nutrients.

On the other side of my image, I showed a meal and dessert from a well-known fast-food establishment: six chicken nuggets; medium fries; zero-calorie soda and an ice-cream dessert. These four items totalled 854 calories (377 less than the snacks). I mentioned the nutritional quality was lower but not non-existent. Fries still contain potatoes, which contain nutrients; it's just that they have other stuff added. Chicken nuggets, though not as optimal as fresh chicken, still contain protein and some nutrients. Lastly, ice cream, heavy in cream and sugar, still contains a small quantity of micronutrients. Here's a comment thread between an Instagram user who replied to the post and me:

THEM: *'Fast food is bad for you though. I don't get this.'*
ME: *'Why is it bad for you?'*
THEM: *'It's processed crap.'*
ME: *'That description means nothing particularly useful.'*
THEM: *'OK, if you want to get technical, it has excessive sodium (salt), fatty acids, and sugar which all contribute to high blood pressure and obesity... and don't get me started on the chicken...'*

The Instagram user didn't realize that the combined total of salt for the fast-food items was just over 1g. The recommended limit per day is around 3g. There was also just over 1g sugar in the fries and nuggets, but when you add the ice cream, it becomes 33g in total. The flapjacks, nut bar, nuts and smoothie contain 62g sugar, nearly double. Regarding the fat, the fast food combined to just 3.2g saturated fat across the fries and nuggets, and 8.7g once you add the ice cream. The recommendation is not to exceed 20g saturated fat per day. The snacks amounted to 26.7g saturated fat.

The user had a valid point that basing our diets on whole foods rich in nutrients, protein and fibre is shown across the research to help control body fat and support various health markers. But they failed to realize that moderate intake of sub-optimal foods will not undo the healthful benefits of whole foods. They can also increase overall diet enjoyment, which is a boost for your mental health. Should you eat fast food all the time? Probably not. Should you avoid it entirely if you enjoy it? Probably not either.

This example shows the importance of understanding that sometimes our engrained beliefs aren't reality. Perhaps misinformation, exaggerated headlines, confirmation bias and correlation shaped the views of this social-media user so that they distrusted fast food in any instance. After becoming aware of the finer details concerning both sets of foods and appreciating their impact in overall diet over time, I hope these dogmatic beliefs were held a little bit more loosely.

Jumping to conclusions is kind of like believing that just because you once came across a mouldy blueberry, you must discard the entire tub because all subsequent blueberries must be mouldy too. When we dig deeper, we know it's not the case. It's not that the media misinform us. It's that they continue to allow other people to use them as a vehicle to misinform us. The most valuable conclusions are from those who can deliver the burden of proof after weighing up both sides of an argument and accept that there isn't a compelling case if there isn't compelling evidence.

THE CHARLATAN SNAKE PIT
AND THE INVENTION OF FAKE PROBLEMS

The advantage that con artists and scammers often have over those trying to help people using science and honesty is relatability. If you went on a string of dates and had to choose one person at the end, you are most likely to select the person you got on with best. You may feel you have a connection with them or that they cast a spell over you, drawing you towards them. In essence, this emotional reeling in is what a charlatan is trying to do when talking to you about how their particular system or products can help you rapidly lose weight or improve your health. Emotion is a far more powerful way to get you attached to something than mere data.

Because they can't use data to support their claims, charlatans have to first tear down opposing views to appear more credible. Many do this by labelling science as fixed or paid for by Big Pharma or the food industry, despite not showing any evidence to support this. The possibility of conspiracy immediately sparks powerful emotion, and before you know it, you may assume that a baseless rumour must be a stone-cold fact.

Second, they use fear tactics to build on emotion. The very possibility that something might cause harm appears to be more potent than evidence showing something does or does not cause harm. When we have a string of unusual ailments, we've all taken to Google to try to find out what is going on. In the search results, we see a series of potentially worrying conditions that usually alarms us. This fear may result in desperation to believe in voices that promise to fix the imaginary condition we've diagnosed ourselves with.

Using baseless lies to dismantle mainstream science's credibility creates a snake pit where all types of claims and views become relevant. For example, some claim that calories in vs calories out is no longer relevant to fat loss because it's not new science. If you believe this, it opens the door for a mirage of alternative solutions. These might include green tea, MCT oil, slimming creams, low-carb cookbooks, fat-busting shorts, juice diets, detoxes, intermittent fasting plans, food sprinkles, hormone capsules, slimming clubs, vibrating fat-burning machines, carb blockers and fat burners. These are portrayed as logical, legitimate answers to losing weight when the answer is simply that calories in vs calories out has withstood alternative theories' tests over time. Just like gravity, discovered by Sir Isaac Newton in 1687, has.

When we are part of a small group who know things that we feel the masses are too stupid to understand, it makes us feel special. Suddenly, the charlatan has an army of emotionally charged followers going into battle to defend their views at all costs without the need for any evidence. Is it really that people genuinely believe the earth is flat? Or is it just the feeling of euphoria and sense of identity they get from being attached to a theory they think is exclusive to them, no matter what it may be? Do we live in an age where, even though people know they are wrong, they still defend themselves to defend their cult?

METABOLISM MYTH BUSTING

How many times have you seen an advert claiming that the reason you're not losing weight is because your metabolism is too slow or broken? It may be accompanied by an expensive metabolism-boosting supplement, a bunch of science-y words with the promise that it will increase your metabolism, resulting in you burning more calories and losing weight. Surely it's a no-brainer?

Your metabolism is simply the calories you burn. The more weight you have, the more calories you burn at rest, meaning your metabolism is faster. As you reduce your weight, you burn fewer calories at rest, so your metabolism is slower. Therefore, the miracle metabolism-boosting fat-loss supplement is physiologically useless. The charlatans that market it don't understand that your metabolism slows down as you lose weight; it doesn't speed up. Yet they are selling you a product that allegedly speeds up your metabolism and results in weight loss – this is impossible. The idea that a supplement is powerful enough to alter metabolism is also silly. But under the illusion of science, it can appear convincing enough to at least try.

Left unchallenged, we are all at risk of falling into the traps that charlatans and scammers lay for us. If we don't challenge them, our exposure to their exaggerations, cherry-picked pseudoscience, flawed logic and flat-out lies only increases, potentially one day reeling us in. The more we see something, the more we are inclined to believe it. From there, we can become emotionally and financially invested in unproven products, procedures and recommendations that probably won't help us at all, or worse, could be dangerous.

How can I make money?! I know... I'll tell people they have something wrong with them and I have a scientific-sounding solution.

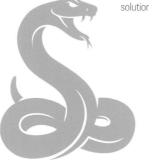

I can't lose body fat and don't know why?!

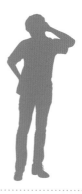

You have a broken metabolism. Here's some pills that will fix it for £100.

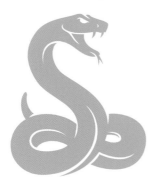

This sounds about right! Here's £100!

PART 2

HOW TO AVOID BEING SUCKED INTO DIET TRIBES

EVIDENCE
IS LIBERATING

A follower of mine sent me a direct message saying that she swapped the 5 litres of soda she used to drink each week for flavoured water or zero-calorie soda, changing nothing else in her diet or exercise regime. She told me that she lost over a stone (7kg) in six months and cancelled her slimming club membership. She said she wasn't aware that such a simple change could have such a huge impact. It reversed years of mental torment at the hands of diet culture. She was liberated, aiming to make more enjoyable changes to maximize further results. Weight loss was no longer a struggle.

For the first time in her life, she understood what a calorie deficit was and how her weight loss was evidence it could be used to her advantage. Considering the body of science was her first step. The second was questioning views that weren't scientific. The third was aligning the science and her personal preferences, making seamless changes, empowering her to take actions that would change her life forever.

In his book *The Irrational Ape,* Dr David Robert Grimes writes: 'Ideas that are not testable are not science... Those ideas that fail to withstand the trials of investigation must be dismissed. The truth that the earth is round has withstood many tests over time. The idea that the earth is flat has not. Therefore, those who argue the earth is flat are merely giving their opinion, not the truth.' The same logic applies to weight loss and nutrition. We need to be able to investigate, test, avoid biased opinions and apply sound reasoning to our conclusions in order to find the truth. Let's take this concept into part 2 of this section and analyze some of the most popular fat-loss methods. Do they stand up to the trials of investigation?

We need to be able to investigate, test and avoid biased opinions in order to find the truth.

WHY BIOHACKING
IS BOLLOCKS

A self-proclaimed biohacker who claims he will be able to live until 180, also claims on his website that he lost 45kg (100lb) in two years by eating 4,000–4,500 calories per day (likely a calorie surplus) with no exercise. As he puts it, why waste time on sleep and exercise when you can accomplish vast weight loss and look great by cutting out toxins and eating high amounts of saturated fat?

What this man said his body did and what his body actually did is open to debate. He is entitled to believe what he likes, of course. But let's invite our friend evidence-based science into the room. It would argue that he lost 45kg (100lb) in two years because he created a calorie deficit, whether he believes it or not. It would also say this had nothing to do with eating high amounts of saturated fat or cutting out undisclosed toxins.

Due to it being quite tricky to test, claims about the anti-inflammatory benefits of the high-saturated-fat diet also remain unproven when compared to a healthful diet including all foods in moderation. But it's one thing to make a claim that isn't supported; it's a whole different ball game when you argue the complete opposite of what the science says. In communicating the supposed 'health-promoting' qualities of this type of diet, he strongly asserts that consuming large amounts of butter (predominantly made up of saturated fat) in your morning coffee is health-promoting, referring to it as a quality fat that will benefit your health, help you lose weight and live longer. This simply isn't true.

SATURATED FAT
FAKE NEWS

In a television interview in June 2021, the same British actress we discussed earlier (see page 64) mentioned that she put coconut oil in her coffee every morning. She said she did this for two reasons: firstly, fat was the brain's preferred fuel source. Secondly, supplying the brain with fat would fill her up all morning, resulting in less overeating. She went on to say that she ate bacon and eggs every day for this reason too.

Let's dissect this. Like butter, coconut oil is calorie-dense and made up entirely of saturated fat. Contrary to what the actress stated, fat is not the brain's preferred fuel source; carbs are.[27] Fat may well fill us up, but what if the carbs contain fibre to fill us up too? Or what about the filling nature of protein? The actress was instructing us to put a calorie-dense food in a low-calorie drink to lose weight and suggested we should eat high levels of saturated fat every day to benefit our health.

While glorifying the benefits of coconut oil without citing any evidence, she claimed that, by removing vegetable oils, she was able to function better, metabolize food, and then get rid of it, presumably meaning it wouldn't be stored as body fat. To date, there isn't any scientific evidence that supports any of these claims. However, there is strong data in the form of a systematic review which concludes that regularly consuming vegetable oils instead of saturated fats helps lower cholesterol and prevent heart disease.[28] Saturated fat found in butter and coconut oil does the exact opposite, meaning that eating lots of it (as the actress recommended) increases the risk of heart disease.

These statements were not only anecdotal and hypocritical but also dangerous. Her words no doubt resulted in swathes of people following her advice to lose weight and improve their health, only to make weight loss harder and maybe even increase their risk of heart disease. In a short five-minute TV interview, a wildfire of misinformation and non-truths was set alight.

SATURATED FAT
FACT CHECK

Saturated fat is usually solid at room temperature. Foods high in it are the likes of butter, cheese, fatty meat, coconut oil and cream. Eating lots of these all the time is thought to raise what's known as low-density lipoproteins, or LDL cholesterol, potentially leading to an increased risk of a cardiac event later in life.

A meta-analysis of 395 metabolic ward experiments concluded that the higher your saturated fat intake, the higher your LDL, which increases your risk of cardiovascular disease.[29] A recent Cochrane systematic review with more than 56,000 participants found that cutting down on saturated fat led to a 17 per cent reduction in the risk of all cardiovascular diseases, including heart disease and strokes.[30] The same review found that replacing high levels of saturated fats with poly- and monounsaturated fats and starches reduced this risk significantly. Saturated fat isn't harmful per se, but the sheer amount could be if consumption is high over long periods. For example, putting 20g coconut oil in your coffee every day uses up your entire 20g recommended limit of daily saturated fat intake before you've eaten anything else.

It doesn't stop there. Dr Danielle Belardo MD, a cardiologist based in California, had a 39-year-old patient who spent years on a high-saturated-fat ketogenic diet, drinking daily butter in their coffee in order to improve their health and satiety. For context, an LDL level of less than 100 is good; 100–129 is acceptable as long as there are no underlying health conditions; 130–159 is high; 160–189 is very high, and anything above 190 is considered extremely high. This patient's LDL cholesterol was 200, and they suffered an acute heart attack. Dr Belardo noted that although genetics may have played a role, diet also did. She pointed out that this patient was advised by self-proclaimed 'biohackers' that LDL cholesterol didn't matter, and that eating and drinking relatively large amounts of butter and other saturated fats were beneficial to health. But this advice goes directly against the body of scientific evidence and has no rigorous science to back it up. The body of evidence clearly shows that consuming high amounts of saturated fat not only doesn't benefit health but is potentially detrimental to wellbeing.

Outlandish claims that ignore science and recommend precisely what the science doesn't are not limited to biohackers and their outlying army of believers. They surface everywhere, from the deepest, darkest corners of the internet to the front page of your newspaper, or even from your close family. All telling you that their theories will make you healthier and leaner. It's one thing if the claim does not affect health either way, purporting to cure a series of made-up conditions. But it's another to keep claiming it even if it is shown to increase the risk of poor health significantly.

In order to find the truth, we need to let the body of evidence do that for us, not social media posts or bestselling books telling you to put slabs of butter in your coffee every day and eat copious amounts of grass-fed steak to improve your energy levels, burn fat and clear brain fog. Butter, steak and any other food high in saturated fat are not inherently detrimental to health. But, if eaten excessively over time, the risk to your health is undeniable. Lobbing slabs of butter in your coffee every morning to improve your wellbeing or reduce your waistline could end up, over time, doing the exact opposite.

Saturated fat isn't harmful per se, but the sheer amount could be.

DIET CULTS
VS DIY

Hardcore football fans will zealously berate the referee for awarding a free kick to the other team despite there being a blatant foul. Die-hard diet camps appear to operate similarly. Whether it's low carb, fasting, anti-sugar, keto or slimming clubs, followers of each faction all seem to have a blind loyalty to their chosen camp that stretches beyond reason. While each of the aforementioned diets can be used to lose weight if you enjoy them, they aren't necessary. Fortunately, evidence is here to show us why.

In 2018, the International Food Information Council (IFIC) published a survey examining consumers' food behaviours. The survey found that 80 per cent of people came across conflicting nutrition information, and that 59 per cent of these people went on to doubt their food choices. Alarmingly, only 17 per cent believed calories from all sources impacted weight, instead believing the likes of carbs and sugar were to blame. Just 22 per cent of those with a college degree indicated the relevance of calories for bodyweight.[31] By 2020, 30 per cent of those with a college degree believed sugar was most likely to cause weight gain when given the option to say all calorie sources were the same. (Interestingly, the figure was just 22 per cent among those without a college degree.[32])

The 2018 survey also showed that a third of people followed a specific diet, including low carb, intermittent fasting, paleo and keto, with weight loss being the number one motivation for following that diet. By 2020, 58 per cent of people in the survey aged 18–34 reported trying a specific diet, again with their top motivation being to lose weight. That's a lot of people following specific diets...

An estimated 45 million Americans go on specific diets each year and spend a staggering $33 billion on weight-loss products. With so many opting for these popular diets to lose weight, are these restrictive methods any more effective than basic calorie control? Let's consult the body of evidence and find out...

THE LOW-CARB CULT

The idea of reducing carbohydrate intake to lose weight has only become popular in recent decades. But its origin dates back to the early nineteenth century and Jean Brillat-Savarin, a French lawyer and politician who first claimed that carbs make you fat. What evidence did he have to back this up? Well, his logic was that carnivorous mammals that never ate carbs seemed to avoid getting fat and that human beings who ate starches and flour did get fat. Brillat-Savarin's belief chimes with the murky logic of correlation (see page 89).

Since then the low-carb movement has evolved from demonizing starches and flour to arguing that sugar is also a catalyst for increasing obesity rates. If claims about carbs making people fat were made by a French lawyer around 200 years ago, why have they gathered huge momentum over the last decades? And why do some qualified medical and nutrition professionals today still believe carbs cause obesity?

The answer is that these beliefs stem from pseudoscience – a collection of beliefs alleged to be scientific, but which are actually exaggerated or reliant on confirmation bias and an unwillingness to look at the complete body of evidence. For example, some may argue that carbs make you fat because they don't fill you up, resulting in you eating more. This line of rationale may show some carbs aren't filling, but it doesn't prove that carbs inherently make you fat. Even if carbs are less filling and you overeat them, becoming overweight would still be down to eating too many calories, not too many carbs. There are also many additional variables involved, such as how hungry you were and your conscious choice to eat more or not. Neither of these has anything to do with carbs.

The insulin hypothesis

Very low-carb diets like the keto diet have become popular fat-loss interventions. This diet is a spin-off of the Atkins diet and generally only allows its followers to eat 30–50g carbs per day while advocating high fat intake to enter ketosis, a fat-burning state. Put into context, a 50g slice of bread contains around 20g carbs and a medium banana around 30g. Insulin is released when we consume any food to regulate blood sugar, but more of it is released when we eat carbs as they are essentially all varying strands of sugar. Given that insulin is part of fat storage, you might assume that the higher the amount of insulin secreted, the higher the body fat, and the less insulin secreted, the more fat-burning. But this isn't strictly true.

To enter ketosis (the alleged fat-burning state), you can barely eat any carbs and must eat high amounts of fat. This is where the confusion lies. Lots of fat is burned, but it's actually just the dietary fat eaten, not body fat. The amount of body fat you have will be defined by your balance of calories in vs out, regardless of whether these come from carbs or fats. So while insulin helps you store body fat, the amount of body fat you store depends on the number of calories you eat across all food groups and burn through the combination of your BMR, digestive process and movement.

According to the most ardent keto followers and low-carbers, high insulin response over time makes us fat. Thus, we must limit carbs as much as possible and eat more protein and fat. But I wonder what they'd say to the study that compared insulin responses to different foods. The research found that insulin response was the same for white fish (which contains lots of protein and no carbs) and white rice (which contains lots of carbs and virtually no protein). Furthermore, they found that steak, primarily rich in protein and fat, often lauded as the perfect ketogenic food, produced the same insulin response as white bread, a predominantly carb-based food.[33] Another study found that dietary protein increased insulin response in type 2 diabetic patients.[34] Most research does show that the higher the carb intake, particularly sugar, the higher the insulin response, but not increased storage of body fat. Regardless of insulin, the total amount of calories consumed across protein, fat and carbs matters more.

Another study compared the keto diet to a high-carb diet where insulin levels would be much higher and found that participants lost more body fat on the high-carb diet.[35] If insulin makes us fat, how could this be? This research indicates that the amount of insulin secreted isn't necessarily connected to the quantity of body fat stored or an inability to lose body fat.

Keto supporters will claim an array of single studies back their claim that ketogenic diets are superior for fat loss, but remember the importance of looking at all the evidence. A literature review of all relevant studies between 1921 and April 2021 found that ketogenic diets don't appear to have any superior fat-loss benefits for obese individuals or athletic populations compared to non-ketogenic diets when energy intakes are equal.[36] If you enjoy a keto diet, carry on. But to lose fat you still require a calorie deficit.

REVERSING TYPE 2 DIABETES

Some people claim that type 2 diabetes is caused by eating too many carbs or too much sugar. But that's not inherently the case. Type 2 diabetes occurs when your pancreas can no longer secrete insulin normally when your blood sugar is raised after consuming calories. This usually occurs because the visceral fat that surrounds your organs has increased to a point that it impairs the functioning of your pancreas. The more overweight you are in general, the higher chance you have of developing type 2 diabetes because your visceral fat is likely to be high. Thus, the greatest preventative measure you can take to avoid being diagnosed with type 2 diabetes is to avoid becoming overweight.

Quite often, professionals will administer low-carb or keto diets to type 2 patients. This isn't a bad idea as they will reduce blood sugar spikes. But the single most effective way to potentially reverse type 2 diabetes is to create a calorie deficit that will reduce body fat and, crucially, the visceral fat around the pancreas and other organs to help them function better.

The low-carb placebo

Some who attempt to lose fat on low-carb diets report fast results. Does this mean that they work? Well, kind of. But only because they are essentially a method that creates a calorie deficit over time. If you eliminate an entire macronutrient in the form of carbs, there's a good chance you'll reduce the number of calories you eat. Does this make it necessary? Absolutely not.

Others may report quick weight loss or look visibly leaner after a few days of low-carb dieting. But this is just a reduction in water weight. For every 1g carbohydrate stored as glycogen, around 3g water is stored. By cutting carbs, you're also cutting water weight, not necessarily body fat, unless you're in a calorie deficit. You can eat carbs, still lose fat and avoid gaining fat.

In 1975 a study was carried out where obese participants consumed 95 per cent of their energy intake from carbs in the form of rice, fruit and juice. Over a while, participants lost an average of 63.9kg (141lb).[37] If carbs make us fat, how did this significant weight loss happen? The answer is because participants were in a very aggressive calorie deficit at the same time. Though steep calorie deficits are not advisable, this clearly shows that eating carbs doesn't make you fat, and that eating carbs doesn't stop you from losing it either.

Enjoy all macronutrients

A systematic review and meta-analysis categorically showed that carbs were not more fattening than any other food group. It found that when calories and protein were eaten in the same amounts, rates of fat loss were almost identical in low-carb and low-fat diets. Additionally, that marginally higher energy expenditure resulted in greater fat loss in low-fat diets, though this was too small to be noteworthy.[38]

The overwhelming evidence suggests that banning carb-based foods you enjoy in order to lose weight is unnecessary. Furthermore, carbs are rich in fibre, which can help you feel fuller and prevent major illnesses such as colon cancer. Fruits and vegetables are primarily made up of carbs and contain vast amounts of micronutrients to support your overall health, plus they taste superb. You'll often hear people refer to things like pizza, bread, pastries and cookies as 'carbs', and they aren't wrong, but a large proportion of the energy from these foods actually comes from fat. The truth is that most foods contain protein, fat and carbs; enjoy them all. You won't regret it. I promise.

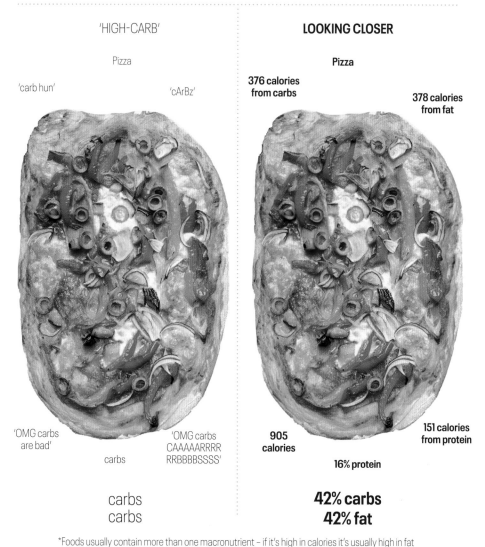

'HIGH-CARB'

Pizza

'carb hun'   'cArBz'

'OMG carbs   'OMG carbs
are bad'   CAAAAARRRR
         carbs   RRBBBBBSSSS'

carbs
carbs

LOOKING CLOSER

Pizza

**376 calories
from carbs**

**378 calories
from fat**

**905
calories**

**151 calories
from protein**

16% protein

**42% carbs
42% fat**

*Foods usually contain more than one macronutrient – if it's high in calories it's usually high in fat

THE GREAT SUGAR PILLAGE

How many times have you heard the following?

'You need to cut out sugar from your diet if you want to lose weight and be healthy.'

Sugar is first and foremost a source of energy. It is also a form of simple carbohydrate. It is found in a variety of foods, from fruit and milk, to cakes, biscuits and sweets. It's not particularly healthful, but just because it doesn't contain many nutrients or provide many health benefits, it doesn't automatically make it harmful.

Those who continue to demonize sugar do so by coming to hypothetical conclusions that aren't connected to what the body of science says. Opposite is an example of how easy it is to twist the science into an anti-sugar narrative:

Sugar is first
and foremost
a source of energy.

1. Is sugar filling? No. This can now be used to claim that anyone who eats sugar will not feel full, assume they will always eat more than they need and get fat.

2. Does sugar contain many nutrients? No. This can now be used as a vehicle to claim that because sugar offers no nutritional benefits, it must cause harm.

3. Is sugar present in many processed, high-calorie foods that taste great and are easy to overeat? Yes. This can now be used to claim that eating in caloric excess is the fault of sugar. Sugar is the scapegoat – and eating it can now be synonymous with being overweight.

4. Does a diet high in processed, sugar-containing foods with hardly any nutrients increase risk of disease and obesity? Yes. Sugar can now be spoken about as an ingredient that increases the risk of disease and obesity. Some may go a step further and claim that sugar causes disease.

But once we take a step back, look at the evidence, remove any underlying bias and critically appraise these sweeping statements, the following must be considered:

1. Does this mean sugar makes you fat? No. Two systematic reviews found that body fat wasn't defined by sugar intake. Instead, an overall calorie surplus over time, indicating over-consumption of protein, other carbohydrates and fats was the key factor.[39]

2. Does this mean sugar causes disease? No. A systematic review concluded that sugar was not responsible for the onset of any cardiometabolic disease.[40] Onset of disease results from several genetic, environmental, behavioural and dietary variables. Depending on the nature of these, sugar may or may not increase the risk of incidence over time.

The above serves as a stark reminder of how easy it is to manipulate the science. But it also demonstrates how simple it is to shut down pseudoscience in a very matter of fact, reasonable way.

Anti-sugar zealots

Suppose sugar did all the terrible things the anti-sugar zealots say it does. Given that fruit and vegetables contain sugar, does this mean we shouldn't eat these low-calorie, nutritious foods to aid fat loss and support health?

If the zealot answers 'no, you should eat fruit and vegetables', then their original statement has already been debunked. But they may come back with something iffy like: 'naturally occurring sugar is more nutritious than refined, added sugars and helps weight loss because your body can process them better'. This statement is simply a fallacy and another example of the appeal of nature – that something is always better in natural form, no matter what. This is why you often see words on food packaging like 'made with natural ingredients' or 'free from x, y or z'. Sugar is a nutrient-sparse energy source, void of nutritional quality.

WHY SUGAR DOES NOT MAKE YOU FAT

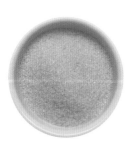

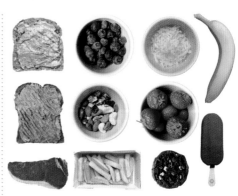

100g sugar	100g sugar within consumed food
400 cal	3,022 cal
	*Hint: 2,622 of these calories aren't sugar

Applying the context of calories in vs calories out as the determinant of fat loss, maintenance and fat gain, 100g sugar equates to 400 calories. But 100g sugar within the foods we eat equates to many more calories. In this example, the overall calories accumulate to 3,022; 7.5 times more calories than the sugar alone. That's the issue. 3,022 calories from food results in excessive calorie intake, not 400 calories from sugar.

Whether it goes by fructose present in mango, sucrose in a cookie, or high-fructose corn syrup in a breakfast cereal, it is broken down and metabolized by the body in the same way.

Remember what I said earlier about there being no good or bad foods? The same applies here: there are no good or bad sugars. For example:

100g fresh mango =
14g sugar (fructose)
+ 66 calories
+ many micronutrients
+ 3g fibre

45g cookie =
14g sugar (sucrose)
+ 205 calories
+ very few micronutrients
+ next-to-no fibre

50g bran flakes
with 200ml semi-skimmed milk =
14g sugar (high-fructose corn syrup)
+ 280 calories
+ moderate micronutrients
+ 7g fibre

The overall ingredients determine a food's quality, not the just the type of sugar it contains. A food high in sugar can also be high in other things, like nutrients, fibre, calories, specific macronutrients or micronutrients. This is why you don't see many people demonizing mangoes for their sugar content in the way that they demonize cookies for theirs, despite being similar in some ways. The 'natural' fallacy may lead us to conclude that refined or 'unnatural' sugar must be worse. But the sugar is the same in the mango and the cookie; it's the other ingredients and their quantities that make the food more or less healthful. Understanding this provides you with a brick-wall defence against morality and self-loathing creeping its way into your sugar-inclusive food choices.

The logic of sweeping anti-sugar crusades claiming sugar is harmful, or poisonous if eaten in any amount, is the same as someone believing that just because the bus was 10 minutes late one day, all buses will be 10 minutes late every day. Thus, on subsequent days they arrive at the bus stop 10 minutes late and miss the bus each time. All because they failed to apply context to the situation.

Just because I'm saying it's OK to eat sugar-inclusive foods, even those with refined sugar, it doesn't mean I'm saying that *all* you should eat is sugar, or that you shouldn't pay attention to the amount of sugar you consume. A high-sugar diet can contribute to being overweight often because its unfilling nature may lead you to eat more and more calories. But this isn't a reason to ban it completely.

You don't have to be for or against sugar. You can sit firmly in the middle, remaining mindful about its inclusion in your diet. Will a moderate portion of food containing only sugar (such as sweets) fill you up? No, that's unlikely. But will a moderate portion of food containing sugar fill you up more if it has relatively high protein or fibre? Yes, more likely. But both options are possible in the context of your overall diet. Not least because the meals you eat either side of the sweets may be nutritious, filling and calorie-controlled.

Something doesn't add up

While diet tribes label sugar as the number one scapegoat for causing the increase in obesity rates around the world, there is another problem with this theory: while obesity rates have been rising, our sugar consumption has been decreasing.

In the early 1960s, 10–15 per cent of the US population was classed as obese. By 2001, this number rose to 25–35 per cent, and by 2014 it was 35–40 per cent.[41] To merge these statistics with sugar consumption, in 1960 the average sugar consumption per person per year was just shy of 36kg (80lb). By 2001 it was around 50kg (110lb), which supports the theory that sugar may be to blame. But here is where the theory collapses: by 2015, sugar consumption decreased to just shy of 43kg (95lb) per person per year.[42] This is merely an interesting correlation, but if sugar is the primary cause of obesity, would obesity rates continue to rise, despite sugar consumption continuing to fall?

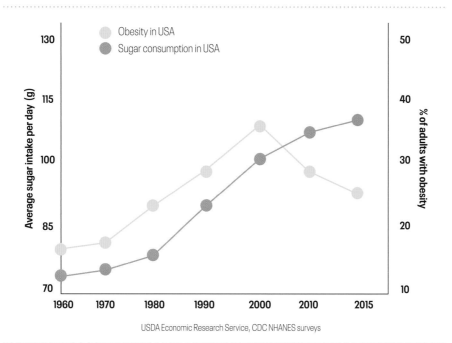

USDA Economic Research Service, CDC NHANES surveys

HOW TO AVOID BEING SUCKED INTO DIET TRIBES

Is sugar more addictive than cocaine?

We've unearthed some pretty convincing evidence that sugar doesn't cause obesity, but what if it is addictive, almost forcing us to eat too much of it, resulting in inadvertent calorie excess? One of the recurring media headlines in recent years is that sugar is as addictive, or more addictive, than cocaine.

This myth largely comes from a study that showed rats preferred to consume sugar-sweetened water than intravenous cocaine; 94 per cent of rats chose the taste of sugar, leading researchers to conclude that intense sweetness surpassed the rewards of the class A drug.[43] The researchers say that this study proves that because some rats still preferred sugar, despite being addicted to cocaine, sugar must be more addictive than cocaine for humans. You can see why the press had a field day and why so many nutritionists and dietitians were hooked by the sensational discovery. But how reliable was this study?

'DON'T EAT THAT!
SUGAR MAKES YOU FAT DAMMIT!'

**LET'S TAKE A CLOSER
LOOK SHALL WE…**

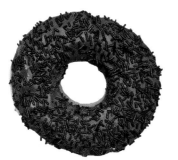

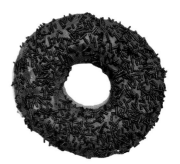

'It's pure sugar
and it'll turn
straight to fat!!!'

**230 calories
8g sugar (32 calories)= just
13.9% of this doughnut is sugar**

Answer: not very. Rodent research is notorious for being inconsistent. But not only that, this study argues that if a person was addicted to cocaine but selected sugar instead of it on occasion, they must be addicted to sugar. This completely neglects the possibility that those cocaine addicts may also eat sugar. After all, it is food, and food is needed to survive. I'm pretty sure that those suffering from cocaine addiction still eat sugar and are still addicted to cocaine. The two are not mutually exclusive.

If sugar was truly addictive, why aren't people eating it straight from the bag? How many people do you know who do this? Instead, we tend to go for combinations of sugar, fat, salt and additional flavours that we enjoy the taste of, aka food. By arguing sugar is addictive, we'd have to argue that fat, protein, starch, salt and all additional flavours in the food are also addictive. Sugar on its own isn't overly appetizing, but sugar combined with fat, salt and other flavours is a different story. Take chocolate, cookies, doughnuts, cakes and chips as an example. These foods need much more than sugar to be delicious.

A recent study showed that ultra-processed high-fat foods were more likely to be linked with addictive-like eating behaviours than their high-sugar counterparts. Pizza, chocolate and crisps were the top three foods identified by participants as being hard to control.[44] Though 50 per cent of the energy from chocolate comes from sugar, the fat content is still around 30 per cent. The pizza and crisps both provide over 50 per cent of their energy from starchy carbs, with minimal or no sugar included. To compound these findings, unprocessed foods containing sugar like fruit were much lower down the list than high-fat items like bacon and cheese.

Food causes obesity, but only if we eat too much of it

Over the last few decades, the rise in availability of hyper-palatable, ultra-processed, calorie-dense foods that taste delicious has undoubtedly contributed to growing obesity rates. But once again, only if we overeat them. Instead of blaming sugar, shouldn't we look at the fact that we are more exposed than ever to delicious high-calorie foods that we enjoy the taste of?

Imagine a bridge, a moving car and sugar. A bridge will fall down, but only if a thousand times the traffic it was engineered to hold is placed on it at one time. A car will eventually stop moving, but only if you stop putting fuel into it. Sugar will make you fat, but only if you eat so much of it that it puts you in a calorie surplus. But what if the bridge experiences the traffic it was designed to hold? Or if the car is refuelled? What happens if sugar is eaten, but in moderation? Understanding this context can silence those who slam sugar and help eliminate feelings of guilt when you eat it.

A BRIEF WORD ON INTERMITTENT FASTING

Supporters of low-carb diets often couple their approach with intermittent fasting for weight loss. The latter is essentially time-restricted eating (TRE). Perhaps the most popular model, 16:8, instructs people to fast for 16 hours with an 8-hour eating window. Usually this means you skip breakfast and eat between 12pm and 8pm.

But is intermittent fasting effective for weight loss? Well, given you're reducing the amount of time in the day you're allowed to eat, it could result in a reduction of calories consumed. But as we've already established, you need to be in a calorie deficit if you want to lose weight. There is no evidence showing that intermittent fasting at specific times works better for weight loss than eating at any time you please. If you like skipping breakfast, do it. If you don't, you don't need to. It can be an effective tool, but science says it makes no difference compared with traditional calorie restriction, eating when you like.[45]

Some supporters of intermittent fasting claim that having long breaks between eating increases the reformation or cleansing of cells. This is known as autophagy, leading to improved health. Is this true? Yes. But let's invite context into the room to get a balanced conclusion. A literature review found that although fasting increases autophagy, so does general calorie restriction.[46] This is strong evidence to suggest that long periods of fasting don't improve your health any more than eating regularly. In any case, suppose you stop eating at 9pm, fall asleep at 11pm, wake up at 7am and immediately eat breakfast. That's 10 hours without eating anyway. Is waiting an extra 3 or 4 hours before you eat really going to make that much difference?

A bridge holding the amount
of traffic it was designed for

A bridge holding 100 times
the traffic it was designed for

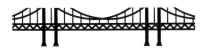

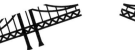

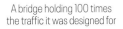

it stands

it collapses

A car with fuel

A car that runs out of fuel

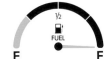

½
FUEL

E   F

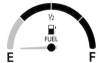

½
FUEL

E   F

it moves

it stops moving

Moderate/low amount of high-calorie, sugary foods
consumed each week:

High amount of high-calorie, sugary
foods consumed each week:

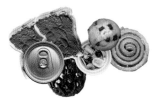

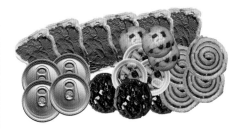
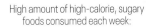

1,750 calories
*Sugar is enjoyed and calorie intake is moderate – no problems

6,500 calories
*Excessive calories become the problem, not sugar

HOW TO AVOID BEING SUCKED INTO DIET TRIBES

THE SLIMMING CLUB LOCK-IN

As we know, you need a calorie deficit to lose weight. So, you'd think communicating this would be the first bit of help that slimming clubs give their new members. But this isn't the case. In fact, this advice is usually nowhere to be seen across their websites, blogs and other marketing tools.

Additionally, they seem to replace scientifically useful terms and measurements, such as calories and energy balance, with their own terms that group foods into made-up categories. Ultimately, these mean absolutely nothing. Within this jargon are foods that you can apparently eat in unlimited amounts and still lose weight. Telling members that they can eat unlimited quantities of these foods and still lose body fat is problematic, mainly because many of these 'free foods' are calorie dense. Following this advice could easily result in members not being in a calorie deficit, or worse, eating more calories than before, resulting in weight gain – the exact opposite of what they want. Is this because they are discouraged from understanding what a calorie deficit is, and how many calories they are eating?

Foods high in calories are often labelled with words that can evoke feelings of shame, or sin. While members are encouraged to track these foods, the slimming club has already stripped all useful information from them. Surely it is more logical to be aware of calorie values? Or protein? Or total calorie intake? After all, connecting these simple scientific terms with your behaviour is incredibly useful in making informed decisions and understanding if you're adhering to a calorie deficit for weight loss.

DO THE SCALES REALLY MEASURE 'SUCCESS'?

With most weight-loss attempts, success is measured by weighing less over time. For many, this involves privately weighing themselves and recording progress along the way. However, some slimming clubs do things slightly differently. They weigh you every week in public alongside other members, oh and you have to pay for it too. Is this what losing weight is about? Public embarrassment if you haven't hit your target?

In any case, the scales you step on to measure weight loss are not as accurate as you might think. As well as body fat, the bit you want to lose, each time you step on the scales you're also measuring muscle, water, food, organs and if you're wearing them, clothes. Some of these things can fluctuate day to day and week to week.

If you eat carbs or salty foods, you are more likely to retain more water weight, adding to your total weight. If you resistance train, you may build more muscle mass, increasing your total weight too. Your weight can also change depending on what stage of your menstrual cycle you're at. Therefore, over short periods, you could lose body fat, but gain weight that isn't body fat, then step on the scales and believe you've failed. In contrast, you could gain a small amount of body fat, but eat fewer carbs and salt, resulting in a total reduction in your weight, even if it wasn't fat loss.

Instead of turning up week in week out with your self-worth hinging on a slimming club consultant telling you what your entire mass' relationship to the ground is, isn't there a more accurate, motivating short-term measurement? Slimming club consultants issue failure and success based on a number they don't fully understand. Ultimately, this weekly number doesn't measure fat loss as accurately as you're led to believe, nor have any relevance to your self-worth. Success surely cannot be based on a single number. How happy are you? Do you enjoy your food? How do you look? What exercise PBs did you achieve? How do you feel? These are the questions skilled and empathetic coaches ask in order to help, not simply saying, 'Better luck next week'.

A long-term solution or short-term deception?

In July 2019 I received a message that alarmed me. A follower of mine sent the following:

'I had no idea that "free foods" were full of calories... I've been part of a slimming club for the last 3 years and I've stayed the same weight. Loss... gain... loss... gain... I have this week started to count calories and have stopped my slimming club... I have a lot of weight to lose, but I know I will get there now.'

In August 2021 I received the following:

'I went for the first time at 13. It's set me up with so many bad habits. I'm 27 now and still the same weight I was years ago. I'm trying to learn to hate myself less and unlearn so many problematic behaviours.'

Another message read:

'I was told by a slimming club consultant I should be losing between 4 and 7lb every week. I felt like I was failing when I didn't do that.'

Perhaps the most concerning message I received said:

'I was persuaded by my slimming club consultant to become a consultant. I wanted to help people, but soon realized it wasn't about helping people or learning about nutrition at all. It was mainly about how to get members and how the more members you get, the more money you make. I was penalized if a member didn't lose what the slimming club suggested they should and was taught how to have a dig at the member, making them feel rubbish in the process. I remember each new year I'd see the same people knowing my consultant just saw pound signs, not compassion.'

Clearly, there will be opposing stories to rival these to demonstrate that slimming clubs work for many people, at least initially. But the reason they do is because following them has created a calorie deficit over time, resulting in weight loss. But given members aren't aware of the straightforward reason why they lost that weight, the chances of them putting it back on increases.

SLIMMING CLUB

200g of each:

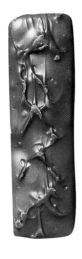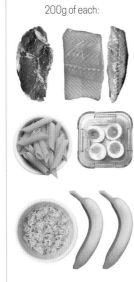

'12 SINS'
(Limit these as
you're being bad)

'FREE FOODS'
(Eat as much as you want
and you'll still lose weight)

'I'm following the plan, so why
aren't I losing weight?'

THE REALITY

200g of each:

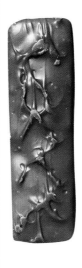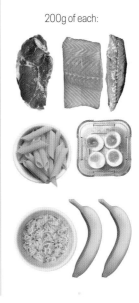

248 cal   **3,332 cal**

(Information that directly relates to calorie
intake – a major thing that defines body fat)

**Because you might be eating
too many calories**

You don't need to count calories to create a calorie deficit, but it can be a useful tool. I was delighted that the penny dropped for the woman who messaged me in 2019. She knew that she needed a calorie deficit, something she wasn't told during her three years as a slimming club member. Think of the time she could have saved, or, God forbid, the situation she'd be in if the penny hadn't dropped? If slimming club members tracked their calorie intake, would they still feel obliged to follow the slimming club's weight-loss plan? I have my doubts. Are these eating systems designed to pull the member further away from the science to make them reliant on the slimming club instead? Are the clubs creating their own set of rules to give the impression that their system is the answer to years of failed weight loss, pain and heartache? I'll let you decide.

The marketing messages from slimming clubs claim that they are allowing their members to stay informed to reach their weight-loss goal. But their eating systems and nonsensical food-labelling jargon often denies their members the information that would allow them to make informed food choices. Entrenching their members in a quagmire of made-up words means that they don't understand the significance of calories, a calorie deficit, protein, fibre and enjoyment over time. Understanding and acting on these is what educates you to make changes and understand why. In contrast, slimming clubs overcomplicate the very simple scientific principle required to lose weight and keep it off.

The nature of the way slimming clubs are often set up makes you reliant on their system, not science. If this is your cup of tea, go ahead. If you want to stay fully informed about the science of losing weight, perhaps don't. It is frustrating that companies continue to claim they are following the science in their plans yet make up their own unscientific terminology that forms the nuts and bolts of their structure. Is there some useful advice on behaviour change? Possibly. Will their plans result in you being in a calorie deficit? Possibly. Will your diet be more healthful? Possibly. Will you be able to stick to it? Possibly. But possibly isn't good enough. You deserve to know exactly how you lose body fat, not least because this knowledge will help you keep it off forever. If you are paying a slimming club each week and you are following the rules they set, but aren't getting the results you want, you have the right to ask your consultant why. Then ask why their rules are required in the first place. What exactly is the point?

THE ANTI-DIET
CONTRADICTION

There are many positive elements to this movement, such as:

1. Rejection of fad/extreme diets
2. Rejection of the idea that if you're overweight, you must lose weight
3. Eating without fear
4. Positive support for those recovering from eating disorders or disordered eating

Naturally, as a trend gains momentum, it gains more followers. With more followers comes more diverse personalities, motives and agendas. This has resulted in many jumping on the train but vandalizing the carriage with claims that are designed to propel the movement, but only serve to undermine it.

'95% of diets fail'

In recent years this statistic is constantly referenced by extreme sections of the anti-diet movement who use it as evidence that intentional weight loss never works. Because your chances of success are just 5 per cent, there's no point trying to lose weight. But how reliable is this statistic?

Well, it originated from a 1959 study by Dr Albert Stunkard. The study had 100 participants and, in Stunkard's words, 'they were just given a diet and sent on their way'. After two years without any support or education, only 5 per cent of participants had lost weight and kept it off, creating the mantra that 95 per cent of diets fail.

Given that it is impossible to gather information on every diet attempt by humans, arguing that 95 per cent of diets fail is bold. Furthermore, this claim is based on research on just 100 people. Does this sound convincing to you? Even Stunkard himself was quoted by *The New York Times* in 1999, saying that 'I've been sort of surprised that people keep citing it; I know we do better these days.'

Numerous studies since, carried out on much larger groups of people, tell a different story. For example, the National Weight Control registry showed that around 20 per cent of overweight individuals successfully maintain long-term weight loss.[47] Is a 20 per cent success rate high? No. Clearly there needs to be more attention paid to the feasibility of weight-loss methods and their sustainability long-term. Still, it does challenge the '95 per cent of all diets fail' myth robustly. We also need to address the emotional aspects of behaviours that drive our dietary choices.

'Being overweight does not mean you're unhealthy'

There is large-scale data to support in broad terms that being overweight increases the risk of certain diseases. As much as this is true, our measuring system for appraising the relationship between weight and health has flaws. For example, somebody could be classed as overweight, therefore at increased risk of a host of illnesses, but depending on where the fat is stored, there will be very different outlooks.

For example, suppose Emily and Lucy have exactly the same body fat percentage. Emily stores a large amount of fat around her abdomen, but Lucy stores much less, instead storing more on her thighs and buttocks.

Our measuring system for appraising the relationship between weight and health has flaws.

Because storing fat around the abdomen increases the risk of poor health, Emily would be at increased risk, but Lucy probably wouldn't be, despite having the same amount of body fat. The fact that Lucy is told she has the same risk as Emily is inaccurate. You can be overweight and be perfectly healthy, just as you can be overweight and unhealthy. It's the same if you're not overweight, too. The problem lies when this important nuance is used by extreme voices to claim that there is no link between being overweight and the risk of worse health.

On one side, we have toxic factions of the fitness community who believe that you must look a certain way to be worthy, pushing their ideology without any thought for what you want. On the other side, extreme factions of the anti-diet movement counter this toxicity by instructing their followers not to lose weight at all. Both fail to listen to what you want. If you want to lose weight because you believe it will benefit your health or boost confidence, do so. If you don't, then don't. What if it will improve your health? Being denied this opportunity seems to contradict the anti-diet mission statement of free will. Your weight doesn't define your self-worth, but you should still be allowed to make your own decisions about it.

In early 2021, a doctor went on live TV in the UK and not only said diets don't work and weight regain is inevitable, but that losing weight also negatively impacts physical health. The data simply doesn't support these outlandish claims. I can't help but feel that extreme narratives such as this one are reactions to personal traumas suffered from extreme fad diets. If this what they think losing weight involves, no wonder they are dead-set against losing weight. I would be too. But just because somebody has had a bad experience on a miserable diet, it doesn't give them the right to lob all dieting interventions into the same bag and tar them with the same brush.

If the anti-diet movement is to continue being a beacon for freedom to eat without fear and nourishing mental health, its core founders need to distance themselves from the extreme personalities within it and focus on its strengths.

WHEN GOOD INTENTIONS GO WRONG

Most diet camps feed on the tribalism of their followers. They try to convince you that their method is superior and that you will be special for choosing it. But ultimately, there isn't enough evidence to back them up. They are arguably stripping you of your individuality and pulling you away from the all-important key to weight loss – adhering to a calorie deficit over time, eating what you love when you like.

Deciding you want to lose weight is one thing, but it isn't the most important. Sticking to a calorie deficit over time is. Although low-carb, no-sugar, intermittent fasting, keto or slimming clubs carry huge claims, not one of them will help you shed so much as 1g of body fat if you don't eat fewer calories than you burn. Can they be useful? Sure, if you enjoy them. Are they necessary? No. Their restriction, rigidity and food demonization can often make them difficult to enjoy and stick to long term.

Remember that the media exists to entertain, sensationalize or exaggerate to keep the viewer engaged. Some of what they say might be true, but at other times it may lack crucial context. Questioning claims and asking for evidence is intelligent and diligent. Following something without looking at the evidence runs the risk of investing in something that isn't relevant to your goal and can even harm it.

> Questioning claims and asking for evidence is intelligent and diligent.

It's only natural to be drawn to new ideas, even if they don't seem rock solid. The type of car you have ultimately doesn't matter as much as having any car in the first place. No matter what the car, it will still take you from A to B. The type of house you live in ultimately doesn't matter as much as having a roof over your head. Whether it's a luxury mansion or a cramped one-bedroom flat, both protect you from the cold and bad weather. The type of dieting method you choose to lose fat ultimately doesn't matter as much as sticking to it over time. So, when low carb, keto, intermittent fasting, slimming clubs and fat-loss supplements come calling, claiming they are your only answer, be aware that they might actually make your goal harder to achieve.

I can't help but wonder if all the dieting fads have been created as business opportunities rather than empathetic, logical, lasting solutions to losing weight. Instead of enriching us with tools, they patronize and withhold information we need to get a grip of things ourselves. With fear and confusion, they take advantage of our vulnerability and desperation to lose weight and better our health. Do they care about us? Don't we deserve better?

THE
TAKE-HOMES

One thing diet tribes have in common is that they each portray their system as the easiest, most straightforward answer to effectively losing fat. Ironically, they are anything but. They often over-complicate matters, invent pseudoscience to fit their narrative and simply don't align with what the body of science says.

Low-carb diets may work for fat loss, but only because they eliminate an entire macronutrient, which can result in a calorie deficit over time. But the evidence emphatically shows low-carb diets are not better than carb-inclusive diets for weight loss.

Cutting out sugar may work for fat loss because the high-sugar foods you cut out like sweets, chocolate, cakes and pastries are also high in calories, which results in a calorie deficit over time. But the evidence shows that sugar doesn't inherently cause fat gain more than overeating any other food. It's not filling and perhaps reducing it may lead to better food behaviours, but you can include it as part of an enjoyable diet and still lose weight.

Intermittent fasting may work for fat loss because restricting the time you allow yourself to eat results in eating fewer calories, which leads to a calorie deficit over time. But there is no evidence to show that it is any more effective for weight loss when compared with a regular calorie deficit, eating at any time you choose. It also doesn't appear to improve your health.

Slimming clubs may work for fat loss if the changes you make to your diet accidently put you in a calorie deficit. But the refusal of these clubs to educate you about this key principle and their seeming willingness to pull you further away from important information you need for long-term success means you are far less informed, potentially making lasting weight loss harder.

Do you need a calorie deficit to lose fat? Yes. Do you need to do any of diets or clubs discussed in this section to lose fat? No. Perhaps this is why these diet tribes continue to ignore the key principle required for fat loss to occur. Once you've understood this, are they still relevant? Perhaps not. You can eat carbs, you can eat sugar, you can eat at times you please and you do not have to join a slimming club. Anyone who argues against this is not looking at the evidence. Adherence to a calorie deficit on your own terms is far more powerful than a specific way of eating that you're unfamiliar with. The more specific the diet, the less room for your preferences to be included. That's not a good thing, trust me. Losing weight long term and being in good health is about including as many of your preferences as possible while creating a calorie deficit over time, with plenty of room for flexibility and enjoyment. My guess is you can do all of this without any specific diet, and you'll be mentally and financially richer for it.

If you genuinely enjoy these ways of eating, or any other rigid eating method, please continue with them. Otherwise, trust what the science says. It arms you with the tools to avoid suspect claims and understand what works and why. This is kryptonite to the charlatans, scammers and pseudoscientists out there and liberates you to make your own decisions based on solid evidence.

The truth is *your* method, *your* mindset, *your* preferences and *your* patience are more powerful than any dieting method. You need to put yourself first. Let's explore how to do this in the following section.

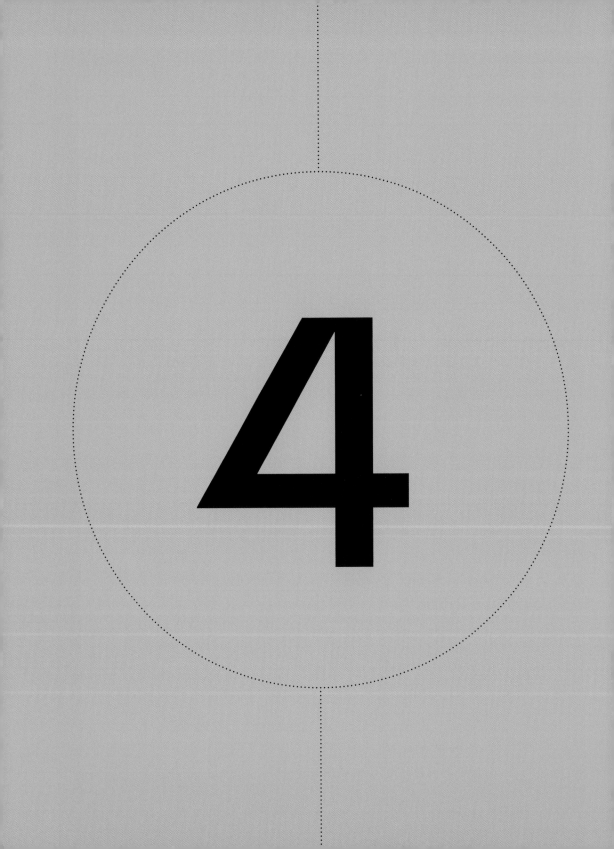

MENTAL STRATEGIES TO STAY ON TRACK

INTRINSIC AND EXTRINSIC MOTIVATION
YOUR WHY, WHAT AND HOW

I first met Ron in March 2015 when I introduced myself to him in the car park of my personal training studio. As we sat down to chat, he cast a nervous, quiet and unhappy figure. Ron was 68, a retired postman of 40 years, newly diagnosed with type 2 diabetes and had had both knees partially replaced. He was also classed as medically obese. Ron had never set foot in a gym, let alone lifted weights before.

Within 12 months, Ron was deadlifting 150kg from the rack, had lost 19kg (3 stone) and all but reversed his type 2 diabetes. Another year on, Ron was celebrating his seventieth birthday by deadlifting 200kg. He had also lost a further 12.7kg (2 stone) and joined a gym to train outside of our sessions. How did Ron achieve these goals at his age, and with his physical limitations? Did Ron and I strategically create the mothership of programmes, culminating in him significantly improving his health, lifting double his bodyweight and losing 31.8kg (5 stone)?

No, we did not. In fact, it was much simpler. Twice a week for a few years, Ron just showed up to our sessions. In the beginning he was quiet and unassuming, perhaps low on confidence. But over time, with each passing session, Ron came out of his shell. I could see how he enjoyed working hard – it meant something special to him and he used to turn up half an hour early. We would chat about football and other sports. Ron would even bring me snacks he'd acquired out shopping and asked me for help when his phone wasn't working properly. As well as being his personal trainer, I was his friend. A bond had been created and it was clear that this once quiet, anxious man was now a completely different person, capable of extraordinary things.

I would love to claim I'm a master personal trainer and expert psychologist for transforming Ron's physical and mental health. But 100 per cent of the physical, mental and emotional benefits Ron experienced were the direct result of his own intrinsic motivations, or motivation from within. His facial expressions constantly showcased his sheer desire to achieve new goals and experience success. He wanted it, needed it and believed he could get it. His main motivation was progression, pushing through barriers and enjoying his own success, not necessarily weight loss. Though the latter clearly benefited his physical health, and he did look much leaner, the only reason Ron and I became aware of his 5-stone weight loss was because he got weighed during his routine hospital check-ups.

From being sedentary for years after his retirement, Ron started moving more and made tiny tweaks to his diet that made all the difference. Ron never set out, nor expected, to lose 5 stone, defy his waning knees or reverse his diabetes in a year. In fact, he didn't set any weight-loss targets at all. Maybe that's why he achieved so much – because there were no limits. Instead, he was immersed in the critical elements required for long-term change – a sustainable, enjoyable process. As long as Ron continued with his daily process and saw gradual improvements along the way, the outcome was inevitable.

Throughout my entire career, Ron is the only client I didn't have a training or nutrition programme for, yet he achieved one of the greatest results. What was I to Ron? Someone to talk to and occasionally give simple pieces of advice he understood and followed. I still keep in touch with Ron, he still brings me snacks and struggles to work his phone.

I also had a client named Rachel. She trained with me on and off for 18 months. She was in her late twenties and desperate to lose weight to transform her life. Her main goal was to fit into a dress she wore years earlier. By this stage of my PT career, I was past overwhelming my clients with as much information as possible to prove my worth, so I made sure I reinforced the basics in terms of nutrition and training. But there were a few problems. Rachel was constantly late for her sessions, sometimes by up to half an hour. Unlike Ron, she complained each time she had to stand up and exercise. She ate chocolate cake for breakfast and didn't take my advice on creating a calorie deficit seriously. I had my work cut out.

Daily choices and habits over time define your outcome.

Despite minimal success, Rachel's goals kept updating. One month she entered a weight-loss challenge at work. The next she started an Instagram account to document her weight loss and hold herself accountable to the world. She even told me she wanted to lose weight, so she'd be able to have a full-length picture on a dating app. She spent a fortune on alleged fat-loss supplements, online meal plans and fitness gimmicks.

I quickly realized that while I gave what I deemed the most useful, relevant advice I could, Rachel would still have to complete 100 per cent of the actions herself. She'd never cooked before. She didn't truly understand how relevant calories were or how to track them. And moving more went directly against her lifestyle habits for the past decade.

Over the weeks and months, there wasn't any progress. Was it my advice? Then it dawned on me that Rachel was possibly paying me to ignore my advice. She didn't trust it. Was I just another fat-loss gimmick she assumed would deliver her the results if she handed over the money?

As time progressed further, the surprising thing is that Rachel was still hugely motivated to lose weight. This was evident in her spending thousands of pounds and months off work attending fitness bootcamps in Thailand and motivational talks in America.

Rachel was an incredibly driven professional. Given that money talks in business, perhaps she assumed that the more she spent on so-called fat-loss fixes, the better they'd work. After all, it was definitely more expensive than my repetitions of calorie deficit, food diaries and increasing steps. Eventually we both decided that it simply wasn't working. It wasn't anyone's fault, but in the years after, I always wondered what it would have taken for the penny to drop. Did she really want to lose weight? Or did she struggle so much because her motivation was extrinsic, trying to please others and fit into what she thought society demanded of her? Did she truly want it for herself? Was she so fixated on the outcome that she didn't appreciate that the process was the most important thing?

Daily choices and habits over time are the things that define the outcome. Was Rachel another victim of the fitness industry's quick-fix fat-loss gimmicks, selling you the world but delivering a flawed, unsustainable process? Only Rachel can answer these probing questions.

Before you decide on doing anything, I want you to ask yourself the following questions:

WHY
Why do you want to lose weight? How will it benefit *you*? Why will it make your life better than it is right now? If you can think of at least one benefit, proceed. If you can't, then you don't need to lose weight.

WHAT
If you have intrinsic motivation to lose weight, what do you need to achieve it? So far, we've established that you require a calorie deficit.

HOW
If you've made it to this stage, it is the all-important part. How do you achieve long-term weight loss?

VISUALIZING
YOUR JOURNEY

Over the course of a flight from London to Singapore, the pilot will make hundreds of tiny changes, altering the aircraft's altitude and direction. Each sophisticated tweak doesn't appear significant – but once they all add up over the course of the 12-hour flight, the aircraft has travelled 6,765 miles, ascending 35,000ft, descending back again and ending up on a different continent. Though we don't necessarily see them as noteworthy, each tiny alteration to the flight path along the way is pivotal to the safety and success of the flight.

This is what happens every time we make decisions that influence how we eat, move and sleep. The tiny turns we take shape the success of our diet, overall health and happiness. Like the flight, just because tiny tweaks might take time to manifest and don't appear to be giving instant results, it doesn't mean that they aren't significant.

Each time you eat, think of it like one minor turn out of the hundreds that an airbus A-380 needs get to its destination safely. We often assume the plane travels in a straight line to its destination, but this isn't true. Perhaps there is a storm on the horizon which means the plane must slightly deviate course. In the case of turbulence, the plane is built in a way that can handle it, ultimately powering through to clear skies unscathed. Just like there is no perfect straight line from one runway to the other, we need to empathize with ourselves and realize that our weight-loss journey may not be perfect, or linear, but we can still get to our destination.

Our assumption is that autopilot flies the plane, not the pilot, and the fat-loss intervention we choose gives us the results. But neither of these are true. Planes were designed by humans, and without humans operating them, they cannot fly at all. The fat-loss intervention doesn't give us results, fat loss cannot occur unless we act, and it cannot continue unless we combine action with enough enjoyment to keep going.

Quite how a 5,000-tonne aircraft can take off, hurtle through the sky at 500mph and land on the other side of the world within 12 hours is a virtue of the wonders of modern engineering and technology. But humans will always be required to steer and deal with potential problems en route. If the captain sets the aircraft's course to fly between London and Singapore, the aircraft will land in Singapore, irrespective of the type of aircraft used or the wind direction.

We cannot change how our bodies function and process our commands. But the condition of your body still depends on the commands you give it. If you eat fewer calories than you burn over time, the end destination is reduced body fat, irrespective of the dieting method used, foods eaten, or exercise performed. If you increase sleep from 5 hours per night to 8 hours, the end destination is greater cognitive function and more energy. If you quit smoking, the end destination is greater cardiovascular health markers.

Your mind decides your beliefs ⟶ Your beliefs dictate your actions ⟶ Your actions are processes ⟶ These processes add up to define your overall outcomes over time.

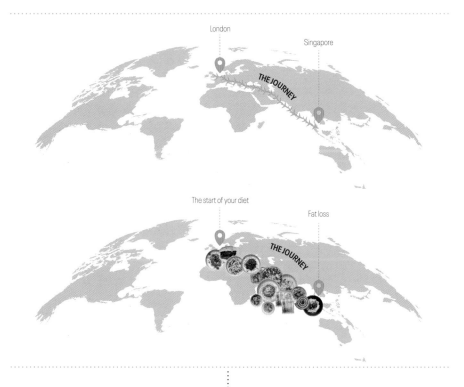

THE CURIOUS STORY
OF THE LITTLE RED DOT

Before the 2010 British Open, South African golfer Louis Oosthuizen was struggling to find form, unable to focus before he hit each shot. In golf, wind, rain, hazards, undulating greens and club selection make every shot completely different from one round to the next. This means focus is critical to decide what to do and execute the plan. Years later, Oosthuizen said in the build-up tournaments to the British Open that 'his head was everywhere'. Unsurprisingly, this was reflected in poor results.

Enter Karl Morris, one of Europe's most highly regarded golf psychologists. He met with Oosthuizen prior to the British Open. In order to help him regain focus before each shot, he adopted what's known as the 'anchoring' technique, developed from 'classical conditioning,' first developed by Ivan Pavlov, a Russian physiologist. It worked by putting a red dot on Oosthuizen's golf glove, something he would see just before every shot. This is how it would work:

1. Think of a time you played a brilliant round of golf.
2. How did you feel when you played this round?
3. What was your mood like?
4. What was the level of focus?
5. Give this state of peak performance a colour.
6. Put a dot of that colour on your golf glove.
7. Before every shot, look at the dot and use it to refocus on what you need to do.

For Oosthuizen, the colour of the dot was red. He looked at it before every shot of the British Open, and he won.

The seven steps above do seem like a lot to mentally absorb before every golf shot, or every meal choice you make. But even if you bear in mind one or two of the points each time, it can help to realign your focus and improve the quality of your decisions. Your anchor doesn't have to be a red dot but having something you see every day can help to remind you why you are trying to make changes in your life and what you need to do to achieve them.

Oosthuizen had all the attributes to win a major golf tournament, but he just needed to be reminded of how good he was. To regain his confidence and clarity of thought to execute each shot. He took 201 shots in total over the tournament, each one accumulated to build his victory. Though some shots didn't go according to plan, the red dot served to put the poor shots out of his mind as he stepped over the next one, ensuring a consistently high level over time. Each time resetting, refocusing and calmly executing. The red dot isn't limited to Louis Oosthuizen. Just a few months later, Graeme McDowell adopted the same strategy, enabling him to win his first and only major tournament.

Because you're human, you will inevitably go over your calorie targets, or skip your exercise. But instead of feeling like you've failed, simply refer to your anchor for reassurance that it doesn't matter. What you do next, over the following hours, days, weeks, months and years count more than a single moment in time. Your outcome is the average of your ongoing processes. When you feel them creeping in, stop guilt and shame in their tracks and refocus yourself on your anchor and your process. This will enable you to see the bigger picture and simplify what you need to do going forward.

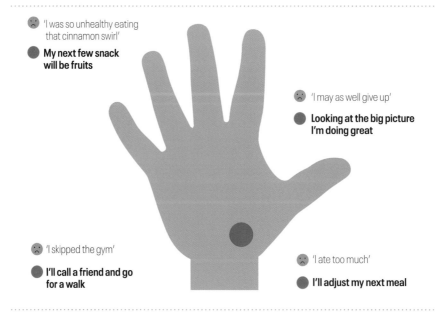

'I was so unhealthy eating that cinnamon swirl'

My next few snack will be fruits

'I may as well give up'

Looking at the big picture I'm doing great

'I skipped the gym'

I'll call a friend and go for a walk

'I ate too much'

I'll adjust my next meal

DIETING - ONE BRICK AT A TIME

Oosthuizen's major victory was built by 201 golf shots, not one. Houses are built of thousands of bricks, not one. A tower of blocks collapses because of all the other pieces removed, not just the final piece. The quality and success of your diet is defined by every meal you eat across your entire life, not one. The point is, all the golf swings, bricks and meals matter as much as each other. They don't have to be perfect; they just need to collectively support your goal over time.

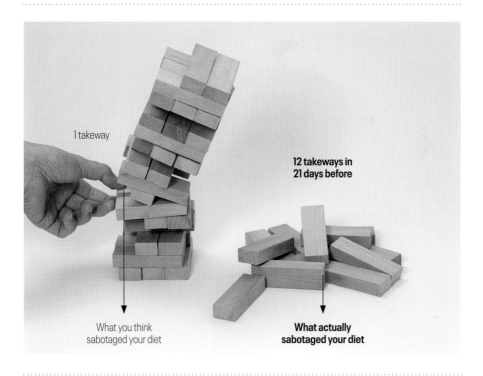

1 takeway

12 takeways in
21 days before

What you think
sabotaged your diet

What actually
sabotaged your diet

PLANT YOUR ROOTS, EXPAND YOUR BRANCHES

Once a tree seed finds the right conditions, the first roots break through, anchoring it and taking in water from the developing plant. Next comes the embryonic shoot, pushing up through the soil. This shoot then becomes a seedling above ground. At this stage it is extremely vulnerable to damage, disease and deer grazing. When the tree grows to over 3ft tall, it becomes a sapling with flexible trunks, smooth bark, but still unable to produce flowers or fruit. When the tree is mature enough, fruits and flowers blossom in the right conditions. When a tree is mature, its roots are its strongest element. Experts believe a tree's roots can be so powerful that they can split solid rock as they grow. From this robust foundation, extensions of the trunk and branches continue to grow, amassing a huge, mighty structure.

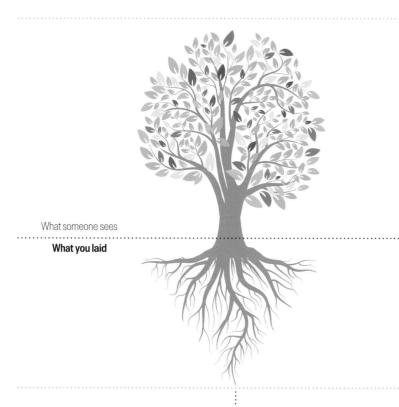

What someone sees

What you laid

Changing your daily habits resembles a growing tree. Over time, your individual behaviours, beliefs, friends, family, social environments, job, sleep and self-esteem will all collectively influence your food choices, physical activity, energy levels and mental health. Your way of life is determined by your habits.

What do you do if you've built a tree of habits that hasn't supported your goals? Let's say you aren't motivated by much, your friends aren't empathetic, your family doesn't support you, your social life has been built on fast food and idle occasions, you have a job you hate, you sleep poorly resulting in low energy levels, you don't enjoy your own cooking and you mentally beat yourself up for making unsupportive food choices over and over again. How can you turn this around?

Well, you have to build another tree. Slowly manifesting growth of the trunk and branches, bit by bit. It requires a conscious focus to change habits but doing it slowly and choosing the easiest options is going to make it much more achievable. It sounds daunting, but I assure you it needn't be.

It requires a conscious

focus to change.

What excites you? What are your friends doing for you? What is your family doing for you? What job would you enjoy? What simple steps could result in better sleep to improve your energy levels the following day? What home-cooked meals do you enjoy? Name one logical reason to feel guilty for eating that pizza. If you can answer these questions, you have the basis to build a new tree of habits. Growing with each process until it flourishes to support a desirable ongoing outcome. What starts out as a seed, turns into the bedrock from which you live your life. Manifesting small victories, one second, minute, hour, day, month and year at a time.

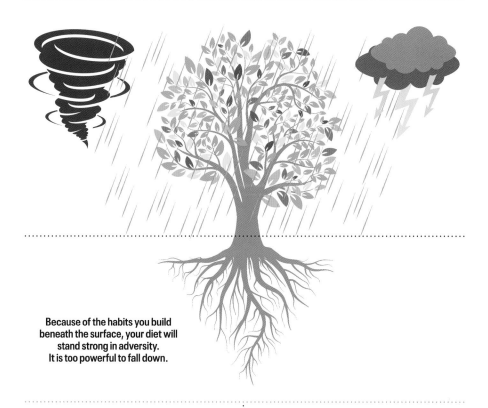

Because of the habits you build beneath the surface, your diet will stand strong in adversity. It is too powerful to fall down.

DO WE MOVE LESS
AS ADULTS?

Domestic cats spend the first 3–4 years of their lives constantly training to fight in order to kill prey – it's what they're hard-wired for. But when they get older, have you noticed you don't have to replace as many ripped-up carpets, shoes and ornaments? This is because, over time, they become adapted, or domesticated, and realize there's no need to fight or kill. If a rodent presented itself, their natural instincts would ensure most cats would re-engage in 'kill mode', but due to the scarcity of these situations, most spend the majority of their time eating and sleeping – and moving less. Unless your cat is overweight, they also usually reduce the amount of food they eat as they get older.

CHANGES IN PHYSICAL ACTIVITY
ACROSS OUR LIFESPAN

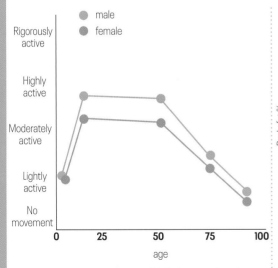

Adapted from K.R. Westerterp (2018), 'Changes in physical activity over the lifespan: impact on body composition and sarcopenic obesity'.

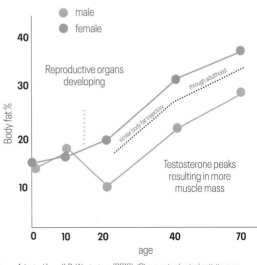

Adapted from K.R. Westerterp (2018), 'Changes in physical activity over the lifespan: impact on body composition and sarcopenic obesity'.

Now think back to when you were a child or a teenager. There's a good chance you moved quite a bit more than you do today. Perhaps you played sports in the park with friends and had to walk to and from school where you did PE twice a week. Due to being too young to drive, perhaps you walked places to meet friends. The most vivid memories you have of these years likely centres around events you had to physically get to.

When we enter our twenties and thirties, are we human versions of domestic cats? Do we settle down as we get older? PE twice a week? Gone. The school sport you participated in? Gone. Walk to school? Now you drive to work. Walk to your best friend's house? Open WhatsApp instead. Unlike childhood, in adulthood most of the important parts of our life are sedentary, so we move less. Perhaps our jobs and finances occupy our time and minds more, resulting in increased fatigue. Perhaps our use of technology means we don't have to move as much as before. All of this suggests that our daily energy expenditure reduces as we get older, certainly when compared to childhood.

HOW TO MOVE MORE

1. Make time for yourself and select an activity you enjoy – even if it's just 15 minutes per day to start with.

2. Write down the time and place to do it. Whether it's a walk, meditation or playing with the kids in the garden. Physically seeing it written down increases your chances of actually doing it.

3. Ask a friend to join you. This means you're not only accountable to yourself, but that you'll be letting your friend down if you don't show up.

MAKE THINGS NEAT

A tonne of feathers weighs the same as a tonne of steel. But there is no doubt that you need a lot more feathers to make up that tonne than you do blocks of solid steel. A single feather is all but weightless. However, if you get enough feathers together, they can accumulate to weigh substantial amounts.

Non-exercise activity thermogenesis (NEAT) stands for all the movements you make outside planned exercise. Whether it be fidgeting, scratching, blinking, talking, cleaning, gardening or walking. All of these insignificant movements form around 15 per cent of your total daily energy expenditure (TDEE). Like feathers, each episode of NEAT is probably so insignificant that you don't even remember it happened.

And that's the point. If a form of moving appears insignificant, it must be easy. We often think that in order to lose weight we need to join a gym, hire an expensive personal trainer or punish ourselves in fitness bootcamps. But the reality is that if you sleep for 8 hours, you have 16 hours to increase your energy expenditure each day.

Some modes of NEAT will be more effective than others. Walking, household chores like washing up, gardening and doing laundry will burn more calories than blinking and talking. This means there is still a degree of decision-making required to use NEAT to your advantage. In one study, they found that increasing NEAT had a huge effect on participants, even those who were overeating by up to 1,000 calories a day.[48]

Technically, walking isn't NEAT as it's regarded as planned exercise. But it's easy to do and doesn't require a great deal of effort, so let's make it an exception to the rule. Walking is a hugely achievable way to

Increasing NEAT is an easy, continuous process, built on habits.

increase your NEAT and you can combine it with listening to music and podcasts. Setting yourself daily step targets means you can chip away at your calorie burn without much effort. Parking further away from the supermarket, taking the stairs instead of the escalator, locating scenic spots and going for a 20-minute walk when your friend rings you are easy ways to increase your step count with minimal effort or fuss. Each step chipping away at your goal, just like each feather chips away at reaching that tonne in weight. Increasing NEAT is an easy, continuous process, built on habits. Compared to planned exercise it is all but effortless, which makes it easy to stick to.

SLEEPING FOR WEIGHT LOSS

In 2018, Wang et al. conducted a study with interesting results. Overweight or obese adults were separated into two groups, one group was to sleep for around 6 hours 20 minutes per night, the other roughly 90 minutes less. The results showed weight loss in both groups to be similar, but of the weight lost, 83 per cent of the weight lost by the group who slept more was fat, compared to just 58 per cent in the group who slept less.[49] This indicates that the better we sleep, the more energy we will burn throughout the day. This doesn't mean we must sleep for 12 hours per day, but that increasing sleep by just an hour per night could end up benefiting our fat-loss goals.

DAILY 1 PER-CENT-ERS

Ron's success (see page 139) was down to 1 per cent improvements compounding over time, resulting in constant improvements in his physical and mental health. He chipped away and kept showing up. He found a set of sustainable and enjoyable behaviours. For fat loss, sustainability is not about having willpower, it's about finding ways to make it easier so that it works, and you stick to your calorie deficit.

In my second book, *Still Tasty*, I asked my followers to vote for their favourite recipes. Unsurprisingly, pizzas, burgers, pasta, fry-ups, lasagne, pancakes, curries and desserts formed most of the votes

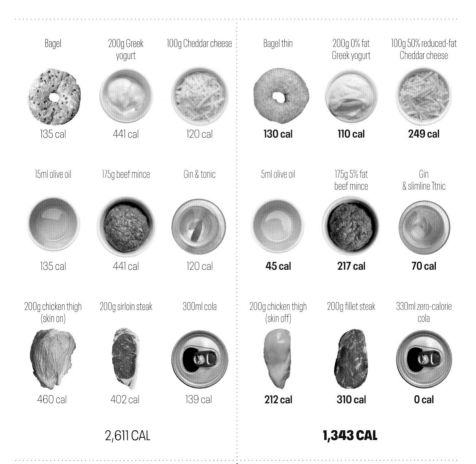

Bagel	200g Greek yogurt	100g Cheddar cheese	Bagel thin	200g 0% fat Greek yogurt	100g 50% reduced-fat Cheddar cheese
135 cal	441 cal	120 cal	**130 cal**	**110 cal**	**249 cal**

15ml olive oil	175g beef mince	Gin & tonic	5ml olive oil	175g 5% fat beef mince	Gin & slimline Ttnic
135 cal	441 cal	120 cal	**45 cal**	**217 cal**	**70 cal**

200g chicken thigh (skin on)	200g sirloin steak	300ml cola	200g chicken thigh (skin off)	200g fillet steak	330ml zero-calorie cola
460 cal	402 cal	139 cal	**212 cal**	**310 cal**	**0 cal**

2,611 CAL | **1,343 CAL**

because, let's face it, they're delicious. However, the fact that all of them contained several hundred or even thousands of calories per portion meant eating them regularly can make a calorie deficit a lot harder to attain. But I quickly realized that I could make these same dishes for fewer calories. It turns out that a lot of these dishes are high in calories because they contain a few high-calorie ingredients. Calories in fatty cuts of meat, hefty portions of cooking oil, cheese, Greek yogurt and cream quickly add up. But fortunately, there are lower calorie alternatives of these same foods at your fingertips.

These daily 1 per-cent-ers aren't limited to easily reducing your calorie intake. As we touched on in section 1 (see page 34), eating enough protein is important for fat loss. Usually when a food has a lower-calorie alternative, they strip a degree of fat from it, meaning that to make up the same weight as the original product, more protein will be present. For example, 200g Greek yogurt contains 12g protein and 264 calories, but 200g 0 per cent fat Greek yogurt contains 20g protein and just 110 calories. Given they taste very similar, that seems like a great deal if you enjoy Greek yogurt and fat loss is your goal.

In a cheese sandwich, swapping 100g regular Cheddar cheese for 100g 50 per cent reduced-fat Cheddar saves 167 calories. Across five cheese sandwiches, that's 835 calories. Over 20 cheese sandwiches, it's 3,340 calories (which equals around 1lb body fat). Let's suppose you like cheese sandwiches so much that you eat 100 every year. By switching to the lower-calorie Cheddar, you'd save 16,700 calories, which equates to 4.5lb body fat. That's a third of a stone, or around 2kg body fat lost by eating the same sized portion of virtually the same food in just ONE favourite eating experience.

Instead of beating yourself up about eating that pizza every couple of weeks, chipping away at your goal with these enjoyable, easy adjustments can empower you to know that you can still enjoy those calorie-dense foodgasms too. Focusing on what is achievable right now instead of getting caught up in the outcome will ensure you focus on the daily processes that compound to achieve your goal.

HIGH-FIBRE FOODS (*PER 100G)

Want to increase your fibre intake to feel fuller and improve your gut health?
Simply fill your cupboards and fridge with high-fibre options.

Raspberries	Blackberries	Pear	Mango	Blueberries
3g (32cal)	**3g** (32cal)	**3g** (47cal)	**3g** (66cal)	**3g** (68cal)

Broccoli	Lentils	Avocado	Wholewheat pasta	Chickpeas
3g (40cal)	**3g** (101cal)	**3g** (210cal)	**3g** (168cal)	**3g** (130cal)

Black beans	Wheat hoops	Wholemeal bagel	Prunes	Cashews
7g (110cal)	**7g** (388cal)	**8g** (250cal)	**8g** (272cal)	**8g** (581cal)

Oats	Wholewheat cereal	Kidney beans	Wheat biscuits	Almonds
9g (374cal)	**9g** (380cal)	**10g** (111cal)	**10g** (362cal)	**11g** (607cal)

Cacao nibs	90% Dark chocolate	Coconut	Bran flakes	Flaxseed
11g (630cal)	**12g** (607cal)	**14g** (633cal)	**15g** (359cal)	**24g** (508cal)

MENTAL STRATEGIES TO STAY ON TRACK

HABIT STACKING
AND PAIRING

In James Clear's bestselling book *Atomic Habits*, he talks about habit stacking. The idea is that in order to introduce new habits, you stack them on to existing ones to make them stick. The concept is as follows:

'After/before [current habit], I will [new habit].'

For example:
'After John gets home from work, he puts on his trainers and goes for a run.'

'After Laura wakes up, she takes food out the freezer to defrost in time for dinner.'

YOUR GOAL

YOUR ROUTINE

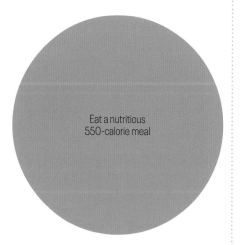

Eat a nutritious
550-calorie meal

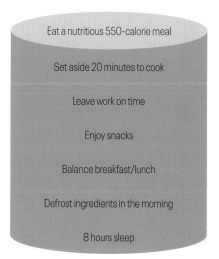

Eat a nutritious 550-calorie meal

Set aside 20 minutes to cook

Leave work on time

Enjoy snacks

Balance breakfast/lunch

Defrost ingredients in the morning

8 hours sleep

'Before Steve brushes his teeth, he turns off the TV in the bedroom to get ready to sleep.'

Attaching something new to something you are already familiar with increases the chances of sticking to and benefiting from the new habit.

Let's say Pete's goal is to drink more water. When does Pete drink more water? At the gym. Therefore, going to the gym will enable Pete to drink more water. Lucy's goal is to cook at least five home-cooked meals the coming week. When does Lucy manage to cook five home-cooked meals? After she goes food shopping at the weekend. Therefore, going food shopping at the weekend will enable Lucy to enjoy five home-cooked meals the coming week. Nicole's goal is to increase her step count. When does Nicole increase her step count? When she arranges to meet her friends in the park. Therefore, meeting her friends in the park will increase her step count.

Stacking and pairing a new behaviour with an existing one means you don't need to make as much effort to implement the new behaviour. If one habit is already engrained, it's the perfect place to stack a new habit that you want to make permanent.

When trying to introduce a new behaviour, James Clear writes: 'Sometimes a habit will be hard to remember, and you'll need to make it obvious... Other times you won't feel like starting, and you'll need to make it attractive... In many cases you may find that a habit may be too difficult, and you'll need to make it easy... Sometimes you won't feel like sticking with it, and you'll need to make it satisfying.'

The secret to creating outcomes that last is to never stop making continuous 1 per cent improvements, combining these tiny advances over time. According to Clear, small habits compound, meaning that the collection of 1 per cent improvements become one powerful cog that is impossible to break. Just like the tree we discussed earlier (see page 148): what starts off as a seed slowly gains strength as it grows into an impressive and powerful tree. Its roots are entrenched in the ground, just as your supportive habits are engrained in your life. Each lower-calorie swap compounds. Each step compounds. Each quality sleep providing you with more energy compounds. Each nutritious meal compounds. Each workout compounds. Each day of happiness compounds.

ZOOM OUT
TO AVOID FAILURE

If improvement is slow, steady and continuous, then failure becomes impossible because you always have more time. Using the flight from London to Singapore example (see pages 143–4), our lives are a series of alterations in one general direction. When we zoom in, some changes may appear devastating at the time, but the further we zoom out, the smaller the alteration looks, enabling us to see the bigger picture of our journey to our destination. As the American author Robert Collier wrote, 'success is the sum of small efforts, repeated day in and day out.'

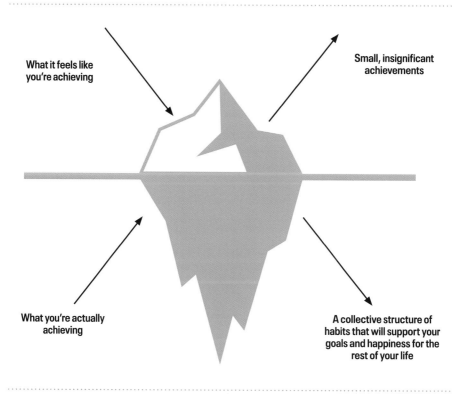

What it feels like you're achieving

Small, insignificant achievements

What you're actually achieving

A collective structure of habits that will support your goals and happiness for the rest of your life

Eating 1,000 too many calories in one day is problematic if viewed through the lens of that single day, but if viewed in the context of a week, a month or a year it becomes less and less significant. It's just one small alteration. It's insignificant because thousands more alterations are required before you reach your destination. In the context of your weight-loss goal, having a takeaway pizza once in a while won't affect your end goal, because thousands more supportive meals await you in the coming days, weeks and months. Time is on your side. No matter what happened on a single day, there is always tomorrow. Practice doesn't equal perfect. Practice equals process, and process equals progress.

'Great things are done by a series of small things brought together.'

VINCENT VAN GOGH

SOMETHING IS BETTER THAN NOTHING

The more insignificant the change, the easier it is to get going. The more you enjoy the change, the easier it is to stick to. The more you zoom out to see the bigger picture, the better idea of progress you'll have. These tiny changes compound to deliver huge differences. This mentality is more sustainable than an all-or-nothing approach (see page 190). The 'all' is intense and temporary, and the 'nothing' doesn't serve your goal at all. Contrastingly, doing 'something' every day, no matter how small, is much more sustainable. It constantly chips away at your eventual outcome, ensuring you're succeeding each and every day.

GET IN THE ZONE

The 'zone' is often referred to as a state of supreme, effortless focus that enables an athlete to perform at the peak of their potential. It is a state of mind that allows cognitive decisions and processes to flow in perfect sync with movements. The present consumes the athlete's attention, and their mind contains the perfect balance of confidence, calm, clarity and execution of skill, which invariably leads to enhanced success. It is the perfect paradox of being focused and relaxed at the exact same time. The result is them successfully achieving their goal while being calmly consumed in the process, not the outcome.

For example, a golfer may need to hole a putt to win the championship. Focusing on the outcome may result in feelings of 'I'm so close to success, but what if I miss...' The brain senses feelings of self-doubt because logic says she hasn't holed every single putt in her career, in fact she's missed many and this could be another miss. This chain of fear impacts her decision-making, routine, confidence and her trust in her ability. The result is a poorly executed putt.

But if her focus was entirely on the process, there's no room left for anxiety. The putt will be hit, and the rest is history. She knows they don't all go in, and that this one might not, but at least she gave it the best possible chance. The possibility of her winning the championship improves by focusing on the present process, not the distant outcome that evokes feelings of elation or possible heartbreak. These emotions are not useful to get the damn golf ball in the hole.

You often hear commentators say that the sportsperson they are commentating on 'must be in the zone' as they serve another ace in tennis, hit another six in cricket or crack in a 30-yarder in football. Though skill, talent and ability are required to excel in sport, why is it that some athletes with the same levels of talent as their peers achieve greater success? And why do some who seemed destined for greatness fail to live up to expectations?

The answer is probably complex and unique to each individual, but ultimately lies in the mental state of the athlete, including pre-existing thoughts, beliefs, motivations and clarity during performance. Self-doubt, fear of failure, overthinking, decision making under pressure, stressful environments, lack of trust in ability or game plans. These all lead people in the opposite direction from the zone, impairing the focus needed to execute the task required for success. In short, unnecessary, useless thoughts at times of stress appear to be the catalyst in preventing an athlete from reaching the heights they are capable of.

The zone is not limited to professional athletes – we can get in the zone too. By informing yourself with evidence-based science, instigating gradual habits, a pragmatic mindset and patience over time, the zone can feel effortless.

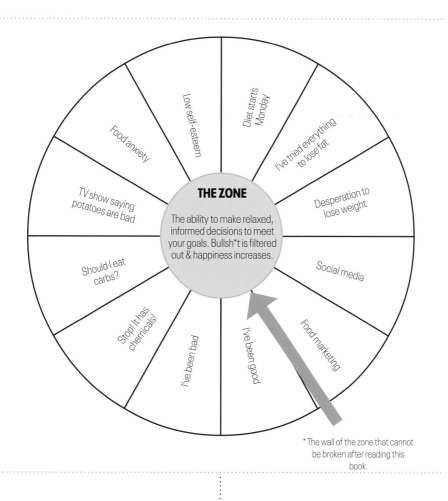

THE ZONE

The ability to make relaxed, informed decisions to meet your goals. Bullsh*t is filtered out & happiness increases.

Low self-esteem

Diet starts Monday

Food anxiety

I've tried everything to lose fat

TV show saying potatoes are bad

Desperation to lose weight

Should I eat carbs?

Social media

Stop! It has chemicals!

I've been bad

I've been good

Food marketing

* The wall of the zone that cannot be broken after reading this book.

Your mind is clear
⟶ You calmly focus on the process, not the outcome
⟶ Ultimately, you develop a state of control without feeling like you have to control anything.

The truth is, there are a lot of similarities between 'the zone' athletes experience and the supportive mental states required to achieve weight loss for good. When making decisions about your diet, you are faced with pressure, noise, rumours, social media and rife misinformation, taking you away from the calm centre of the zone. You don't need perfection, just progress, no matter how small. You don't need to think of food as good or bad, just different. You don't need to completely change your diet, just tweak it. You don't need huge success, just 1 per cent improvements over time. You don't need to struggle, just move forwards.

You don't need perfection,

just progress.

WHY MEAL PLANS
DON'T WORK LONG-TERM

Imagine you are driving a car to a place you've never been to before and the meal plan is your sat nav. You're following directions from the sat nav for the entire journey. You don't know why you're making left turns here and right turns there, but you do so with confidence that the sat nav will take you to your destination. And it's easier than figuring it out for yourself by stopping and looking at a map or consulting the map before you set off. The sat nav may take you to your destination, but once you're there, you have no idea how you got there, or how to navigate from there. What do you do if the sat nav screws up? You're stuck and all of a sudden, you're required to find the route for yourself.

Like my former client Rachel (see pages 140–2), many people think that investing in a state-of-the-art meal plan will automatically deliver the results they crave. If we are unhappy with our weight, we often assume everything about our diet must be wrong and revolutionizing it will snap us back into line.

Most rigid meal plans market their outcome to prospective buyers. 'Eat this meal plan for 30 days and get amazing results...' But adopting this mindset means you fixate on the outcome and ignore the all-important process. Just because the meal plan says you must eat poached chicken salad on Mondays, it doesn't mean you want to. Or even if you did, who's to say on Thursday, when it's next in your meal plan, that you'll feel like eating it? What if you don't want poached chicken salad on Monday or Thursday? What if you don't like poached chicken? What happens then?

According to the meal plan, any deviation equals failure. The meal plan consists of specific foods to be eaten at specific times and the idea that this is the only way to achieve weight loss is simply not true. Why? Because thousands of combinations of varieties of different foods not on the meal plan can still result in a calorie deficit. No food is off limits.

Unfortunately, after deviating from a meal plan, many people believe that they have failed. This simply isn't the case. Individual foods do not determine your weight loss, your balance of calories in vs out over time does. Understanding your energy needs to achieve your weight-loss goal while enjoying a variety of your favourite foods is a more logical and sustainable approach than conforming to a set of rules that restricts your freedom. Instead, eat foods you enjoy at times that are convenient.

Nothing will ever be perfect. Get used to it. We must respect our desire to eat certain foods on an ad hoc basis, balancing them with our goals if we can. If your choice deviated from the ingredients in the poached chicken salad but provided similar calories and nutrients and a more enjoyable eating experience, that's a victory. It also shows the redundancy of a rigid meal plan.

WHAT THE MEAL PLAN SAYS...

WHAT YOUR HEART SAYS...

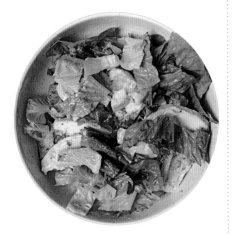

Another boring chicken salad

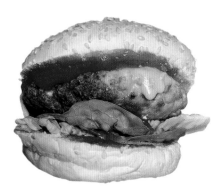

Homemade chicken cheeseburger

460 CAL

479 CAL

*Still on track and the next meal
can be more nutritious

MAKE YOUR OWN RULES

If you do follow through with a prescribed meal plan, what happens at the end of it? You are often left with three options:

1. Continue with the same meal plan, eating poached chicken salad on Mondays and Thursdays forever.
2. Return to your old eating habits that created the issues you are trying to resolve.
3. Pay for a new meal plan that tells you to eat poached chicken on Tuesdays and Fridays.

What about option 4? Instead of feeling like you've failed and giving up, why don't you take control and make your own rules?

YOUR RULES

1
Always select a variety of foods you enjoy but understand the calories in portion sizes.

2
Keep meals simple, varied, convenient and quick to prepare.

3
Keep your fridge, freezer and cupboards stocked with ingredients you enjoy.

4
The night before or in the morning, decide what you'd like to eat for your meals that day.

5
If you think it will help you, make your own meal plan for the days ahead, but realize that you can change it because you're the one in charge.

6
Accept that at times you won't be able to follow your own plan but know you can adjust the following meals. You may have a few days where you have a setback but realize you can carry on.

7
Remind yourself that individual foods or recipes don't inherently result in fat loss but matching your preferences to your calorie needs does.

It doesn't make sense for someone else to decide what you eat and when you eat it. Just like it doesn't make sense trying to fit square pegs into round holes. While the structure of a meal plan can motivate in the beginning, we need to stop believing that someone or something else will achieve our goals for us. We can take on this mantle ourselves and be more effective. Instead of putting our faith in individual foods, we must trust all foods and our ability to align them with a calorie deficit. What if I told you that instead of dropping your favourite chicken pasta dish for a brand-new meal you don't enjoy as much, you don't have to. What if you just need to reduce the cooking oil and change the type of cheese that you melt on top to reduce the calories? Sometimes that's how simple fat loss can be.

FOOD YOU DON'T ENJOY | FOOD YOU DO ENJOY

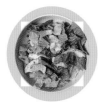

This meal fits my calorie target, but not my tastes

This meal fits my calorie target and my tastes

This meal fits my calorie target, but not my tastes

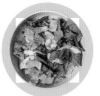

This meal fits my calorie target and my tastes

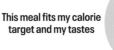

This meal fits my calorie target, but not my tastes

This meal fits my calorie target and my tastes

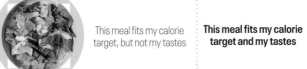

*Trying to grind through food you don't enjoy to reach your goals is like trying to put square pegs into round holes – it doesn't work.

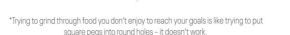

Your success is not defined by how well you can follow a rigid plan to stay on track. It is defined by your ability to be open-minded. Supportive decisions hinge on your ability to be critical enough to discover what information is relevant to you, and how you can use it to your advantage.

In order to achieve big change over time, you must trust small changes. The bigger the change, the harder it is to stick to. If you're privileged enough to be able to make your own food choices, you may as well start making them now. And own them for the rest of your life. You deserve to decide what you eat.

The more you do things, the more they become habits, and the less effort you have to put into them. In order to undo habits that don't serve your goal, you simply need more repetitions of new habits that do. Much like doing reps in the gym, the more you do them, the stronger you get. The more you enjoy something, the more inclined you are to keep doing it. The more time you spend with something, the more you grow fond of it. Over time, each of these scenarios can snowball into an effortless environment where you can work towards your goals at a steady pace, notching up small wins that compound into something special.

Today, we watch aeroplanes fly through the sky without a second thought as to how they came to be. What has become sophisticated engineering of the highest level, likely began by a human watching a bird fly through the sky and asking themselves how it was possible. In around 400 BC, it is thought the first ever flying machine shaped like a bird was able to fly 200 metres.[50] By 1903, the Wright brothers created a manual aircraft capable of controlled, sustained flight. By 1912, the first autopilot was created. By 2005, there was a computerized double-decker aircraft with four million parts, capable of flying 15,000km non-stop. This journey didn't happen overnight. What starts off as an unlikely dream, over time, can compound into something breathtaking. Ask yourself what you want and why you want it. Plant your roots and expand your branches. Each day, bit by bit, chip away, making it easier to keep going and get closer to your goal.

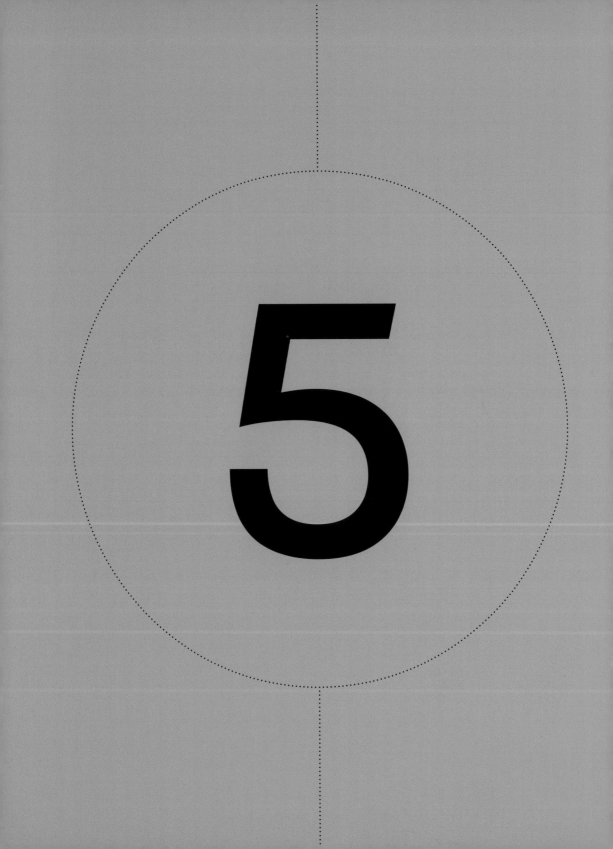

LOSING WEIGHT & FINDING HAPPINESS WITHIN

THE ILLUSION
OF STATUS

We are keen to make ourselves appealing and attractive so that others accept us. This forms our sense of identity. Whether it's meeting a deadline at work, researching a new car to buy or changing our physical appearance to please others, these actions aren't necessary for our survival, but they matter in improving how we look to others.

The illusion of status is not limited to material things – it also applies to our self-esteem. To have an impression of ourselves, we have to evaluate our identity to make sense of it. This evaluation can open the door to ideas of success and failure, positivity and negativity, self-promotion and self-critique. You may buy a new car, which boosts self-esteem. Or you may have to sell your existing car to pay off debts, which reduces your self-esteem. You may buy a big house because you are rich, which inflates your popularity. Or you may have to downsize because your circumstances have changed, resulting in feelings of shame. You may be an ideal weight for your health, which enhances your feelings of self-worth. Or you may be overweight, causing you to believe you don't fit in with what society demands and that you are worthless. These beliefs are simply the illusion of statuses created by your brain's ability to attach emotions to your assumptions.

While your brain can work for you, it can work against you, too. Sometimes, to remind yourself of the reality, you need to keep it in check. Ultimately, an animal's existence is centred first and foremost around finding food and a comfortable place to sleep. If they have that, they'll have a happy, fulfilling life. When you're struggling with negative emotions about yourself, remember that as long as you have food, a comfortable bed and a roof over your head, everything else is comparably insignificant.

STOP
BEATING YOURSELF UP

Our emotions mean that we can make choices which may not correlate with reason or science. We feel the compulsion to think and do things we know present a risk and that are unlikely to reward us. Some of our actions are the result of what we believe will happen or feel has happened.

Here is a list of rational assumptions:

'If I walk into a room with many other people, they are likely to notice me, but unlikely to analyze me or think I look stupid.'

'Eating a single pastry cannot be converted into fat on a specific body part. In isolation, it doesn't contain enough calories to produce a noticeable increase in body fat.'

'Starving and dehydrating myself on the day of my slimming club weigh-in will probably mean I'll weigh less. But this is because of the lack of food and water in my system when I step on the scales, not necessarily a reduction in body fat.'

Here is a list of irrational assumptions:

'I can't wear these clothes; I'll look stupid because I'm overweight.'

'Sheila is right. Ordering that pastry will go straight to my thighs...'

We can trick ourselves into thinking that what is rational isn't true.

'If I starve and dehydrate myself all day, I'll weigh less at my slimming club tonight, and I won't be a failure.'

See what happened there? We can trick ourselves into thinking that what is rational isn't true. The more we let ourselves do this, the more our self-worth is defined by that man on the street who didn't even see us, or the woman who glanced at us on the subway who can't remember us 15 seconds later. These people are mere vehicles for our assumptions about ourselves. If these assumptions are negative, you can become your own worst enemy, robbing yourself of your right to uphold the self-esteem and confidence you deserve. It creates a vacuum of desperation where you believe you must do anything and everything to be better.

We are told by society that we will become better people by losing weight instead of being reassured that losing weight has nothing to do with our worth as people or our value to the world. Losing weight is simply the reduction of existing body fat. It's a physiological alteration. It may potentially make you happier and healthier, but apart from that, nothing else about you changes.

RESIST
QUICK-FIX APPEAL

When you run out of milk, you nip down to the store to get some more before your morning coffee. If you have a burst pipe, you call a plumber straight away to come and fix it. When stuck in a traffic jam, if a shortcut is available, you take it to save time. These are logical solutions that make perfect sense. But what is the answer when you want to lose weight? If you follow the previous examples, finding a solution that provides a fast result is important. Therefore, it makes sense to go on a crash diet. The less you eat, the more weight you lose, right? The only problem is that losing weight takes a lot longer that nipping out for milk, repairing burst pipes or dodging traffic jams.

THE YO-YO DIETING CIRCLE OF HELL

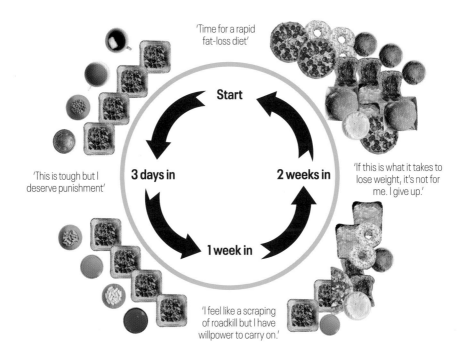

'Time for a rapid fat-loss diet'

Start

'This is tough but I deserve punishment'

3 days in

2 weeks in

'If this is what it takes to lose weight, it's not for me. I give up.'

1 week in

'I feel like a scraping of roadkill but I have willpower to carry on.'

Just as we search for the best plumbers to quickly fix our broken pipes, we assume that searching the internet can provide us with the best solutions to lose weight quickly. This is gold dust to those who seek to take advantage of your vulnerability. Need a new toaster? Order one in 23 seconds and it'll arrive tomorrow morning. You don't even need to move from the sofa. Want to lose weight fast? No problem. Just type 'lose weight fast' into your internet's search engine and you'll find 530 million results. Among others, you'll find juice cleanses, 24-hour fasts, fat-loss supplements, keto powders, appetite suppressants, ultra-low-calorie diets, gruelling DVDs promising six-packs in two weeks and much more. All are based on extreme food restriction and demand you to turn your life upside down. But if you lose a stone in three weeks it's for the greater good, right? How bad can it be? Even if you're miserable for three weeks, you'll have the result you wanted forever, right?

Here's the problem. Even if you stick with the method you've chosen for its limited period and lose the weight you wanted, what happens next? Though it achieved the result, you can't continue on this extreme diet. At this point, you might return to your old diet – the one that caused the problems in the first place. When this happens, the yo-yo dieting circle of hell is born. First you have success in losing weight, no matter how miserable you were. Then you return to your old eating and lifestyle habits for a few months and regain all the weight. Then, like before, you say enough is enough and punish yourself again. You get through it, return to old habits, then diet again a few months later. The cycle goes on and on and on.

GETTING OFF
THE DIETING HAMSTER WHEEL

Metacognition is our understanding of our own thought processes. When looking at weight loss a common thought process is:

'I'm unhappy because I'm overweight.' ⟶ 'I'm ashamed and must punish myself.' **=** 'I must do this extreme diet to lose weight and be happy as soon as possible.'

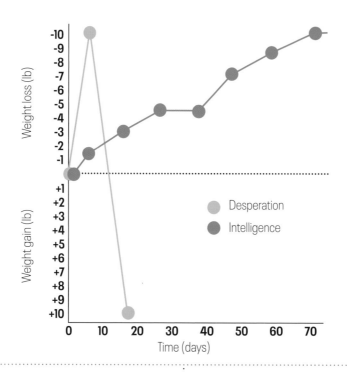

Prioritizing speed is a natural reaction to a desperate situation. If your bathroom is flooding because of a burst pipe, you need a fast solution. If the traffic jam is making you late for a flight, you want that shortcut. But there is an obvious difference between these examples and losing weight. You don't live with burst pipes or traffic jams, but you do live with your body for your entire life. Given that your life is (hopefully) not quick, shouldn't that mean you need a long-term solution instead? One that you enjoy? In order to lose 4.5kg (10lb) body fat in ten days, your life has to be extreme. It's arguably so unsustainable that the only possibility afterwards is weight regain.

Desperation is the willingness to lose 4.5kg (10lb) in ten days. Intelligence is finding enjoyable ways to lose 4.5kg (10lb) in ten weeks. Success is living in a mental state where desperation is replaced by intelligence. Realizing that losing weight is not a race liberates you to enjoy the process. Why does it have to happen so fast? Why does it have to be a punishment? Losing weight is not a mountain you think you need to climb. It doesn't demand willpower or exceptional feats. You don't need kick-starts or self-punishment. Losing weight and keeping it off for good begins in your mind. You need to stop associating weight loss with speed, shame or punishment. Ironically, over time, these are the things that are making it much, much slower.

You need to stop associating weight loss with speed, shame or punishment.

GO SLOW
TO GO FAST

We established earlier that individual foods don't lead to weight gain (see page 51); time does. Because you are always burning calories, it can take months and years before gaining body fat becomes noticeable or problematic. Many report that weight 'creeps' up on them, or that one day they looked in the mirror and noticed their weight gain. There's a clue there. Weight gain is the result of behaviours that occur consistently over time. Logically, shouldn't we expect sustainable weight loss to take the same period? Shouldn't we ignore the idea that losing weight won't take time? Take a step back and think about that for a second. If this statement is plausible, any solutions that promise rapid weight loss must be unsustainable. If it took you years to gain weight, how can you reverse this entire physiological timeline in just a few short weeks?

Let's look at an example. Mandy wants to lose 2 stone (12.7kg) in six weeks. 1lb of body fat equates to approximately 3,500 calories. 2 stone (12.7kg) of body fat = 28lb. 3,500 (calories) x 28(lb) means Mandy would have to reduce her calorie intake by 98,000 calories within six weeks to lose 2 stone. That's 16,333 calories per week and 2,333 calories per day. Mandy is 5ft 7in and weighs 14 stone (196lb). She needs 2,200–2,800 calories per day to maintain her weight, depending on her activity level. The goal is therefore almost impossible to achieve unless she burns large amounts of extra calories through exercise. But given she'd be consuming next-to-no calories, this is nigh on impossible.

Even if Mandy tried to lose the same amount of weight over ten weeks, she would still have to reduce her calorie intake by 1,400 per day, so could only consume an average of around 800 calories if she is relatively sedentary or performing light exercise. If exercise was more regular, she could have around 1,400 calories per day, still a relatively low number. Attempting to eat a few hundred calories per day is likely to cause serious ill-health. Using science to demonstrate what is required for rapid weight loss highlights just how ridiculous and nigh-on impossible quick-fix diets are. Instead of supporting your physical and mental health they are, in fact, detrimental to both.

Usually, desperation means extreme dieting attempts last a few days, but once it is clear that the show cannot continue, the result for many can be feelings of failure, complete curtailment of their goal and a return to ground zero having learned nothing. 'Weight loss is not for me' may be ringing in your ears as you believe you simply don't have the willpower to accomplish it. Each time you attempt an extreme diet and fail, your self-esteem takes another hit. And the yo-yo dieting circle of hell either begins or continues. You hang your self-worth on a number on the scales and are in a constant battle with yourself.

Measuring success based on a number is problematic, but for the sake of this argument, let's compare the above quick-fix dieting attempt to the goal of losing 2 stone, but just 1lb a week. In theory it would take 28 weeks to lose the weight (just over 6 months). It would require Mandy to reduce her calories by 3,500 calories per week, and 500 per day. So instead of a ridiculously low-calorie target needed for rapid weight loss, she could eat 1,700–2,300 calories per day, depending on her activity level. Already it's a lot more sustainable, plus she'll have more energy to move more and increase her daily energy expenditure too. Progress is slower, but it's more sustainable. Although Mandy is going slower, she is actually going faster. Why is this? In short, because she is able to keep going without the need for willpower, and without any feelings of failure.

When you drive a car fast, the speed increases the risk of a crash because you have less time to react. Even if you get lucky in the beginning, the risk remains if the speed stays the same. Going slower is safer because it allows your reactions to catch up when a problem occurs. Just like reducing your speed increases the chances of staying on the road, reducing your speed when losing weight increases the chances of sticking to your diet.

LOSING WEIGHT & FINDING HAPPINESS WITHIN

AVOID 'FAT-LOSS' PRODUCTS

Imagine this: you see a pair of red earplugs for sale purporting a host of noise-cancelling benefits, encased in shiny, colourful packaging. You know the more expensive blue earplugs work well having used them before, but their packaging is boring and dated. Because you believe the noise-cancelling promises are genuine and more convincing, you buy the shiny, red earplugs. Upon use, you realize they don't block out noise at all and barely fit your ears, meaning that you have to go back and buy the reputable pair you know work. Your money and time are wasted.

Let's say the red earplugs represent supplements promising effective fat loss and the blue version represents gradually reducing your calorie intake and moving more. A gradual calorie deficit is at an immediate disadvantage because it can't be sold in a bottle or advertised with grand claims and extravagant marketing. Alleged fat-loss supplements can, making them seem a more exciting and convincing option.

There are two problems here:
1. There's no rigorous scientific data that shows these supplements cause fat-loss on their own.
2. You must be in a calorie deficit to lose fat.

If these supplements don't cause fat loss and you require a calorie deficit anyway, what is the point in taking them? The answer is: there isn't any.

Fat-burner pills are probably the most popular fat-loss supplement, readily available on the high street. But while the marketing cleverly insinuates that popping them will torch body fat like there's no tomorrow, this isn't true. Instead, many of these pills are loaded with caffeine, meaning that by consuming them, you're simply more likely to move more.

REGAINING WEIGHT

Steve and Claire are having a conversation about Steve's weight-loss journey. Steve, who once weighed 18 stone, lost 4 stone within a year by creating a calorie deficit. But over the past three months Steve has regained half a stone. He complains to Claire, 'What's the point of doing this any more?' Claire replies, 'Steve, I understand that it's challenging and frustrating at times, but if we take a step back and assess the past 15 months, you've lost 3½ stone, right? You are happier, have more energy, have improved health markers and can run around with your kids in the garden.' Steve's ears prick up. Claire continues, 'Weight can go up and down and it's never easy to have a constant trajectory in your favour because losing fat is the exact opposite of how your body is programmed – it wants to store it so that you won't starve. The important thing is that you stay engaged and believe in yourself. In the grand scheme of things you've made gigantic steps towards improving your health. Sure, you've gained some weight back, but you know how to lose weight sustainably, so perhaps just take stock and make a few tweaks to get back on track?' Steve replies, 'Well, when you put it like that...'

Claire has successfully reinforced the fact that, over short periods Steve's weight can go up and down, but the average over the long term is what counts. Every time you're disappointed or deflated about gaining weight over two weeks, view that weight gain in the context of the previous two months, or two years. This gives you a more accurate picture of your overall progress.

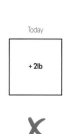

Today

+ 2lb

X

'I've gained weight
so I'm a failure'

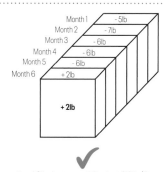

Month 1   - 5lb
Month 2   - 7lb
Month 3   - 6lb
Month 4   - 6lb
Month 5   - 6lb
Month 6   + 2lb

+ 2lb

✔

'I've gained 2lb, but overall I've lost 28lb (2 stone)
in 6 months... Let's just re-assess and ensure
I'm in a calorie deficit...'

THE DREADED
WEIGHT-LOSS PLATEAU

The more weight you lose, the harder it gets to maintain the same rate of weight loss. This is because the less weight you have, the less weight there is to lose. Your body is also hard-wired to store body fat to survive. However, if you're in a calorie deficit, you will continue to lose body fat.

But what if you're convinced that you're in a calorie deficit, but you aren't losing fat? Naturally, this may take you to the dark corners of the internet where pseudoscience lurks, telling you that you're in 'starvation mode' or you have a 'broken metabolism'. Both of these terms are simply jargon made up to sound science-y. What's really going on is that you're simply not in a calorie deficit. This isn't your fault. There is always a rational explanation why you may think you're in a calorie deficit, but you actually aren't:

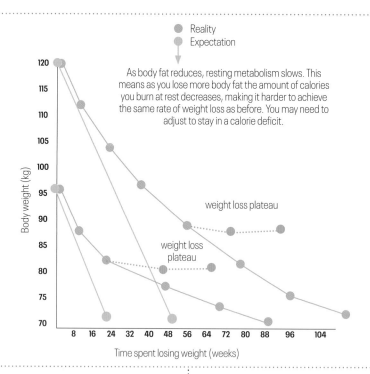

As body fat reduces, resting metabolism slows. This means as you lose more body fat the amount of calories you burn at rest decreases, making it harder to achieve the same rate of weight loss as before. You may need to adjust to stay in a calorie deficit.

Reality
Expectation

weight loss plateau

weight loss plateau

Body weight (kg)

Time spent losing weight (weeks)

WHY YOU MIGHT NOT BE
IN A CALORIE DEFICIT

Underestimating the number of calories you're eating.

You may think you're eating 1,700 per day, but the nibbles here and there that you don't account for take it closer to 2,000.

You are burning fewer calories.

Exercise exertion has reduced because you have less energy. Even things like standing and fidgeting reduce too.

Metabolic adaptation.

If you repeatedly embark on aggressive calorie deficits, your metabolism can adapt so that your BMR, or resting energy expenditure (see page 186), is less than before, causing you to burn fewer calories at rest.

Not reducing calorie intake as weight decreases.

You haven't reduced your calorie intake as your weight decreased to stay in a calorie deficit.

The information you put into the calorie calculator was wrong.

By putting in inaccurate weight, height or activity levels, the calorie target you get may not be the right number to achieve your goal.

WHAT YOU CAN DO TO ENSURE
YOU ARE IN A CALORIE DEFICIT

Go through a period of rigorous tracking for a few days to spot any underestimations or misjudgements.

Log how long you exercise for and the intensity you worked at. Does it match your previous assumptions? Also take note of your NEAT by recording how long you are completely stationary for over a few days.

Ensure you put the right information into the calorie calculator. Each calculator may be slightly different, so try three different calculators and take the average calorie target from all three.

YOU DON'T NEED TO BE
THE BIGGEST LOSER

As you lose weight, your BMR decreases. This means the number of calories you burn at rest is lower than before. On very low-calorie diets (VLCDs), your body needs to adapt more. In the US TV show *The Biggest Loser*, contestants lost huge amounts of weight in rapid time. Six years after the show, 14 of the 16 contestants took part in a study. The results showed that not only had most contestants regained all of the weight, but their metabolisms had also slowed, meaning they were burning fewer calories at rest than they were before the TV show.[51] Previously they were burning around 2,600 calories at rest each day, but six years later, after regaining the weight, the group burned just 1,900 calories per day.[52] According to obesity expert Kevin Hall, 'metabolism appears to act like a spring, the more effort you use to exert weight, the more it stretches out, and the harder it will spring back, regaining and holding onto the fat that was lost'.[53]

YOUR THYROID, PCOS
AND YOUR METABOLISM

There are rare cases where people have an underactive thyroid, causing their metabolism to slow. If you think this may be the case for you, ask your doctor for a test.

Polycystic ovary syndrome (PCOS) is a condition that affects menstrual cycle and metabolism, and the resulting hormonal imbalances make it much harder to lose weight. If Jenny doesn't have PCOS and reduces her calories to 1,800 per day to lose weight, Steph, who has the same activity level, age, height and weight, but does have PCOS, would have to reduce her calories further. It's therefore a good idea for those who have PCOS and want to lose weight to ensure they have a protein- and fibre-rich diet in order to feel fuller.

HOW TO AVOID
SELF-SABOTAGE

If you tripped up and hit your knee on a door, you wouldn't purposefully hit your other knee on the door as well. If your windscreen has a small crack in it, you don't smash the entire windscreen. If you eat three or four biscuits, you don't need to eat the entire packet. So, what if you do eat a few biscuits?

The answer is to eat the biscuits and move on. Your next choice is the most important one. The fact that three or four biscuits are currently making their way into your small intestine is a moment you cannot change. The only option is to move forwards. Getting bogged down in feelings of failure is both useless and nonsensical. You deserve to eat, and you chose to eat a few biscuits on this occasion. Convincing yourself that you may as well eat the whole packet doesn't make sense. It would be the same as throwing away your phone and house keys just because you lost your wallet. In the words of James Clear, 'The first mistake is never the one that ruins you – it's the spiral of repeated mistakes that follow'.

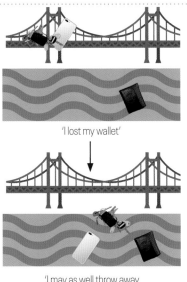

'I lost my wallet'

'I may as well throw away
my phone and keys as well'

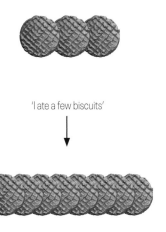

'I ate a few biscuits'

'I may as well eat the entire packet'

THE POSITIVES OF
HOLIDAY WEIGHT GAIN

According to the United Nations, life expectancy around the world is around 72 years on average, though having good genes and taking care of yourself will increase this number considerably. But let's focus on your working life. If you start working at the age of 22 and retire at 65, that's 43 years, 516 months, 2,236 weeks and 15,695 days. Assuming you get the standard six weeks off every year, across your working life that adds up to 258 weeks and 1,806 days. This means that you are on holiday for just 11.5 per cent of your working life.

Whether it's Christmas, a summer holiday or just relaxing at home, enjoy these days. Many of these moments are centred around food and should be cherished. In the grand scheme of things, how much damage can relaxing your diet for just 11.5 per cent of this time do? Instead of worrying about how many calories the pigs in blankets have or abstaining from that extra glass of sangria on a Mediterranean shore, understand that these are moments to cherish, shared with those you hold dear.

If you return home from the best family holiday 4lb heavier, gaining 4lb contributed to one of the most memorable times in your life and was worth it. If you always celebrate New Year 5lb heavier because you've enjoyed your favourite Christmas foods, catching up with friends and family for a couple of weeks, being 5lb heavier contributed to happy memories. Even if your goal is to lose weight, gaining weight over these periods is contributing to a richer, fuller life. When you're 70 years old, you will remember the family meals you ate with loved ones, not whether you made it to the gym four times a week every December. You will smile when you recall the sights you saw with your partner while sipping a beer and indulging in different cuisines, not how many hotel gym sessions you squeezed in or whether your calories and macros aligned. Living life to the fullest means squeezing every last bit of joy out of it you can. Sometimes that means eating roast potatoes, chocolate and loafing around in your pyjamas watching cheesy Christmas movies. You have 88.5 per cent of your working life to be more structured and make supportive dietary choices . There is always time to achieve your weight-loss goal, but moments missed with your friends and family because you were too strict with yourself will never come back.

BE WILLING TO SEE
OTHER ANGLES

It's highly likely that the first time you heard about trigonometry was at school. One day you turned up to school having never heard of it, only to leave that day knowing it existed and what it was useful for. Every building you see is proof that trigonometry has been vital in calculating angles and lengths to make it structurally sound. Suppose when you were young, your parents told you that if you ever became overweight, you needed to cut carbs to lose weight. Suppose this was reinforced for years and supported by the internet when you were older.

In the beginning you knew nothing; you were a blank page. But then when exposed to new information you turn 90 degrees to form beliefs or opinions on that subject. So what if the belief is wrong? Surely reversing 90 degrees will wipe it out, allowing you to start from scratch again? Here's where it gets tricky. In order to allow yourself to change your beliefs, you must be willing to reverse not just 90 degrees, but 180 degrees. In other words, you have to be willing to accept that your beliefs have been completely wrong.

There's no shame in this. We are all wrong about many things, every day. But willingness to accept the possibility that what you have been told isn't completely true will only make you smarter. If you previously lost weight on a two-week crash diet, you may believe that it is the only way to lose weight because you have proof. You were miserable, but you stuck to it. Despite regaining the weight within four weeks, you still believe that crash diets are the only way to lose weight because it's all you've ever tried or believed.

> You have to be willing to accept that your beliefs may have been completely wrong.

WHY THE ALL-OR-NOTHING
MENTALITY IS DOOMED

Suppose you are sunbathing with the intention of getting a tan. You are given two options:

1. You get badly sunburned.
2. You don't tan at all.

You wouldn't select either of these options. What about if you were trying to lose weight?

1. You ban all your favourite calorie-dense foods, stop all social occasions, cook different meals from the rest of your family, force down food you dislike and go to the gym seven days a week.
2. You eat lots of calorie-dense foods, eat takeaways every day, cancel your gym membership and become entirely sedentary.

This is what the all-or-nothing mentality looks like. The risk is that the 'all' is so intense that it simply can't last. The result is that, naturally, 'nothing' has to follow. In order to avoid both of these unsupportive situations, the trick is to always have balance. For example, including some calorie-dense foods in moderation and the odd takeaway is like putting on SPF 15. You're in the sun, but you have a buffer that protects you from its fierceness while still getting a tan.

The trick

is to always

have balance.

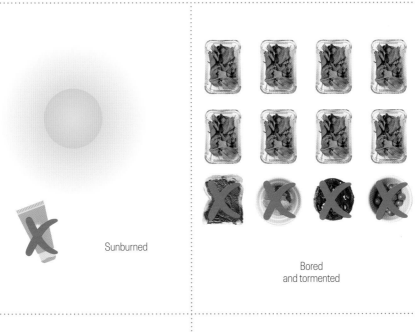

Sunburned

Bored
and tormented

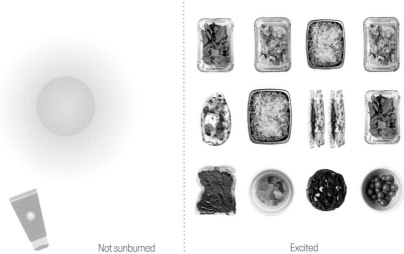

Not sunburned

Excited
and relaxed

LOSING WEIGHT & FINDING HAPPINESS WITHIN

STAY NEUTRAL

Sometimes, it simply needs to be a trade-off between your physical and mental wellbeing. You know by eating a pizza or enjoying a couple of glasses of wine that you won't be supporting a calorie deficit, but you will be enriching your happiness by taking pleasure from foods and drinks you love. You're aware the pizza and wine are calorie dense and not particularly nutritious, but you're also aware of the joy they give you. This must be respected. Ignoring your mental health and failing to accept that you're human can lead to an extreme slippery slope of disordered or binge eating, orthorexia or other eating disorders. You didn't fail when you ate that pizza, drank a few glasses of wine or skipped the gym. You succeeded because you ate and drank things you enjoy, knowing you have tomorrow and many more days to achieve your diet goals.

THE REASONS WE EAT FOOD

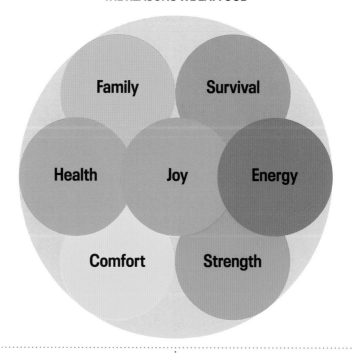

Family

Survival

Health

Joy

Energy

Comfort

Strength

YOU DON'T
NEED TO BE RESILIENT,
YOU JUST NEED
TO BE AVERAGE

Most coaches will praise or admonish your level of resilience for sticking to your diet goal. Praise for avoiding chocolate in the supermarket or ordering a salad at your favourite restaurant, despite preferring the risotto. And admonishment for 'falling off the wagon' and succumbing to a takeaway pizza one weekend. The truth is, when it comes to your diet and eating in general, focus doesn't exist. You can't focus on everything you eat for your entire life – it's not conducive to happiness, it is conducive to obsession. Averages, over time, define your results, not individual choices in single moments.

No single eating choice determines success because there is another choice to make in a just few hours' time which is just as relevant. Over time, all your choices combined create an average. This average is shaped by the momentum of your behaviours, habits and mental health. The trick is to keep an eye on which way your momentum is going. Over the course of a week, what did your diet look like on average? Did you consume enough fruit and veg? How many takeaways did you eat? What was the average amount of calories you consumed? What does your overall diet look like after two weeks, two months or two years? Did that single pizza you ate on 15 February really ruin all your progress? Of course not, so stop beating yourself up about it.

You can't focus on everything you eat for your entire life.

Even if you ate one takeaway a week for a year, assuming you eat three meals per day, the takeaways amount to just 4.8 per cent of your total meals and 14 per cent of your total dinners for the year. You aren't losing focus by ordering a takeaway pizza once a week, which results in you going over your daily target by 650 calories. It's a food you love, and if split over seven days, the 650-calorie surplus can be cancelled out by consuming just 93 calories less over the subsequent seven days. To give an example, this is the equivalent of asking the barista to swap the whole milk in your morning latte to 2 per cent milk for a week. You didn't fail when you ordered that pizza, but if you think you weren't resilient enough, the chance of self-sabotage or apathy increases.

Calmly focusing on averages allows you to see how your diet holds up over time. The data frees you to eat any food at any time without misleading feelings of euphoria, or useless feelings of guilt or shame. Reassuring yourself that this holds true allows you to meet nutritional triumphs and disasters calmly and confidently. Then, in the words of Rudyard Kipling, 'you will treat those two imposters just the same'.

SHAPE
YOUR MOMENTUM

Sports teams experience shifts in momentum when they go on winless runs or a hit a winning streak. Commentators will often say things like 'When you're on a winning run, luck goes for you', or 'When you can't buy a win, the luck goes against you' or 'no matter how hard they try, it just isn't happening for them'. The latter indicating that although effort is still high, positive results are not forthcoming.

Over time, effort and luck have nothing to do with the success of a sports team, or the success of your diet. It's not that fat loss isn't for you or that your friends can lose weight but you can't. Whether it be fat loss, or improving nutritional quality, the end result is entirely down to averages shaped by you. These are influenced by the momentum of your beliefs, actions and habits.

There are always reasons why you succeeded. Just like there are always reasons why you aren't getting the results you want. But trust me, it's not because you enjoy a cookie at work at 3pm every day. It's down to your overall momentum not quite moving enough in the right direction. If it isn't, admonishment and punishment is not the answer.

Instead ask yourself: which way is my momentum going? This requires you to identify where you may need to intervene. For example, if you realize you regularly overeat or are always hungry, you have identified an issue. From here, you can take logical steps such as preparing more satiating meals with more protein- and fibre-rich foods you enjoy, reducing the likelihood of overeating. Suppose you spend an hour on social media each evening and always end up too rushed to make dinner, resulting in ordering several takeaways every week. Setting an alarm on your phone to get off social media after 30 minutes gives you time to prepare more meals that support your calorie deficit.

These are the building blocks of sustainable change. Instead of telling yourself, 'I'm going to do it this time', or 'I'm going to be good today', you are replacing words that don't relate to your goal with actions that directly support it. Actions speak louder than words, always. Once you see that your actions are supporting your goal, it serves as motivation to confidently carry on. These small interventions don't require the intense focus that the fitness industry perpetuates in its advertising. The truth is, chiselled bodies are the result of years of dedication, rigidity, sacrifice and genetics. Instead, small, intelligent tweaks serve as timeless, achievable, impactful interventions that shift your momentum in the right direction. It is the lack of intense focus that makes them more sustainable long term.

ALLOW YOURSELF TO HEAL AFTER TRAUMA

When we become overweight, we have simply adopted habits, behaviours and momentum that have manifested in a consistent calorie surplus. A series of often small changes that occurred over time. Sometimes we are aware of them, other times we are not. While it can be easy to create small changes to reverse the situation, it's important to realize the power of trauma. Deeply emotive events such as the death of a loved one, the break-up of a long-term relationship or other misfortunes have an extremely powerful impact on us. When we deal with these emotions, they take up space that other things otherwise would. Telling someone to simply eat less after they have gone through a harrowing ordeal is as nonsensical as it is unempathetic. When healing is required, nothing else is. Sometimes it will take a few weeks, other times a few months, or longer. In the event that you believe you have healed, but can't seem to get your mojo back, ask yourself how you felt, what your daily behaviours were and what habits you had before. You deserve to be happy and in good health.

IT'S NOT A MOUNTAIN,
IT'S A BUMPY BIKE RIDE

Sometimes losing weight can appear like you are standing at the bottom of a mountain that never stops getting higher. Each time you experience a setback or something important happens, causing your efforts to be postponed, looking up at a seemingly never-ending summit can convince you that it is impossible. So why not instil an alternative image? What if the mountain is replaced by a flat path and you are riding a bicycle instead of trekking upwards? Sure, there may be the odd puddle to swerve, pothole to avoid and you may even get a puncture, causing you to pause for a while. But you're moving forwards, not upwards. It won't always be a straight line, but that doesn't matter. The day we realize that losing weight isn't an uphill struggle, but a simple series of behaviours is the day we might stop struggling for good.

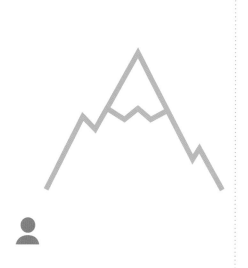
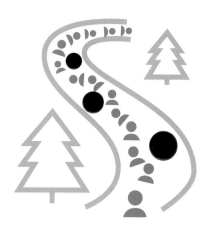

THE SUCCESS LAG

Phil Knight was a student and middle-distance runner at The University of Oregon in the late 1950s. In 1964, he created his first running shoe company called Blue Ribbon Sports. During the following years, the same company faced many ups and downs, being forced to find brand-new factories and company names and struggling to stay out of debt. In 2020, 56 years after Phil Knight's first company was formed, the company it evolved into was valued at $35 billion. Its name is Nike.

For Phil Knight, the fruits of his efforts manifested around 20–30 years after he started his company. There were times when many others would have given up, but by having the courage to carry on, he paved the success of a company that transcends sports brands today. Just because you've been trying to lose weight for a few weeks and nothing seems to be happening, stick at it. Results might be just around the corner, giving you the encouragement to continue. In the words of Winston Churchill, 'success is not final; failure is not fatal: it is the courage to continue that counts'.

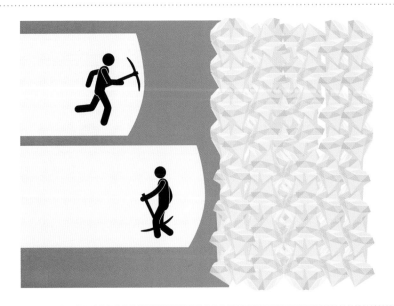

BODY DYSMORPHIA

The next time you're a passenger in a car, make a point of looking at the wing mirrors of the cars that drive by. Focus on them and I guarantee it will make the cars passing by look entirely different. Now the sleek 4x4 looks like it has strange ears sticking out. The thing is, the wing mirrors, or strange ears, were on every 4x4 you admired previously – you just didn't see them. This also happens when we look at our bodies. You focus in on microscopic elements of your physical appearance without seeing the bigger picture. This can cause us to have a dysfunctional, dysmorphic opinion of how we look, compared with the reality. When you see ugliness, fatness and imperfection, others will see beauty, attractiveness and perfection. We need to be kinder to ourselves.

WHAT YOU SEE	THE REALITY
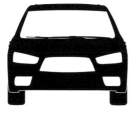	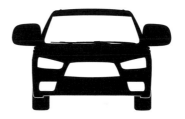
A distorted view of a car	**A car that looks like it has ears**

WHAT YOU SEE	THE REALITY
UGLINESS	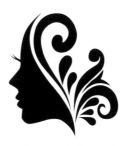
A distorted view of yourself	**Beauty that many find attractive**

WHY FOOD IS YOUR ALLY,
NOT YOUR ENEMY

Regardless of all the various ways we describe food and the emotions we attach to it; we need to eat it to stay alive. We must recognize food as a necessity, just like oxygen and water. It allows you to move, to think. And crucially, it is there to be enjoyed. Even chocolate and ice cream can serve as sources of nutrients to some degree. After eating them you should feel pleased, content, satisfied and calm. You've eaten them and now you're moving on with your life. Without food, you wouldn't exist. Are there healthful sources of food that will enhance various aspects of your overall health? Absolutely. But remember that the next time you beat yourself up for eating 'a little too much ice cream', doing so doesn't benefit you in any way. What's done is done. What you do next matters most.

This is why companies who sell appetite suppressants must be challenged. The products are usually based on flimsy science to satisfy marketing agendas, but this reductionist thinking fails to understand that even if these products did suppress your appetite, resulting in you eating less, you still need to eat. While these companies demonize eating food, you will always need to continue eating if you want to remain alive.

What you do

next matters

most.

Research has shown that appetite suppressants in the form of pills, sachets, weight-loss teas and coffees are abused by around 50 per cent of people suffering with eating disorders.[54] A study spanning fifteen years, analyzing young women in the USA, concluded that the use of appetite suppressants and similar products can be dangerous and is a potential warning sign that the individual may have or is developing an eating disorder. It even recommends public health professionals should create initiatives to prohibit access to such products because of the strong evidence that suggests they play a role in causing eating disorders.[55]

Unfortunately, as it stands, anyone can buy these products, and they are even on sale in supposed health shops, albeit at extortionate prices. These companies perpetuate life-threatening conditions for their own greed, often using social-media influencers to promote products to their young, impressionable followers. If you or anyone you know is suffering from an eating disorder, please seek urgent professional help.

WE NEED BODY FAT

In early 2021, I woke up one morning to the following message from a brave 18-year-old woman in my private Facebook support group, 'The Fitness Chef Community.' It read:

'The family I grew up in has made me believe that I will only be beautiful and accepted if I am thin. And that food, instead of representing freedom and strength, should be restricted in order to achieve looking a certain way. Thus, I have been restricting food, then binge eating since 2017. I want to change my unhealthy mindset and start from self-love, not from restrictions and the fear of being fat.'

Without body fat, we wouldn't be alive. Our ability to store body fat is one of the main reasons humans have survived for so long. Tens of thousands of years ago, when food was scarce and other species died out, we had enough reserves to survive. Body fat, or adipose tissue as it is clinically referred to, is a central metabolic organ that not only enables us to store energy to use later, but also cushions and insulates.

Cellulite is the result of the distribution of fat cells, along with other connective tissues, resulting in fat pushing closer to the skin to create an uneven or dimpled surface. This mainly occurs in women and is more likely to occur in those who have more body fat. A quick google of the word will yield a mass of results detailing how you can treat, prevent or even cure cellulite. Websites sell expensive lotions, but no cream that you rub on your skin can change the internal biology beneath it. Those who say it does are crooks. Cellulite is completely normal.

We must not fear fat. If having more fat makes us happy, we must respect our happiness. Losing fat should be your choice. If you believe you'll feel better and be happier with less fat, then lose fat. But no matter what, your weight will never define who you are. Your past and future thoughts, emotions, beliefs and feelings define you. Ultimately, they will be the things that leave a mark on the people you know and the world you live in. Nothing else.

MAINTAINING THE BODY YOU WANT
AFTER WEIGHT LOSS

In a meta-analysis of 29 long-term weight-loss studies, more than half of the weight lost was regained after two years, and in a further five years more than 80 per cent of weight lost was regained.[56] Further evidence suggests that weight management programmes which focus on maintenance after weight loss tend to demonstrate better long-term maintenance of weight loss compared with those geared towards weight loss only.[57] This research suggests it is difficult to maintain weight loss, and also that focusing on losing weight without a long-term view makes weight regain more likely. So, what do you do once you've reached a size you're happy with?

The key to avoiding weight regain is simple. You just need to consume and burn approximately the same number of calories each day over time. This is a continuation of the habits and behaviours you have already built to lose weight, only now you won't be in a calorie deficit, you'll be eating and moving to maintain your current size. If you lose weight gradually and combine it with an easy and enjoyable day-to-day life over a period of time, you have already built lasting habits. Therefore, there is less chance of you developing brand-new habits causing you to regain the weight you lost. To be sure, it might be useful to use a calorie calculator to work out your maintenance calories. You can use mine for free at www.fitnesschef.uk, then select maintenance as your goal and track them for a few days or weeks. If at any point along the way you regain weight you didn't intend to, resetting the calorie calculator can be a good eye-opener. Otherwise, it's likely you can stop tracking calories altogether once you become astute at eyeballing portion sizes. Remember, calorie counting is a temporary education, not a life sentence.

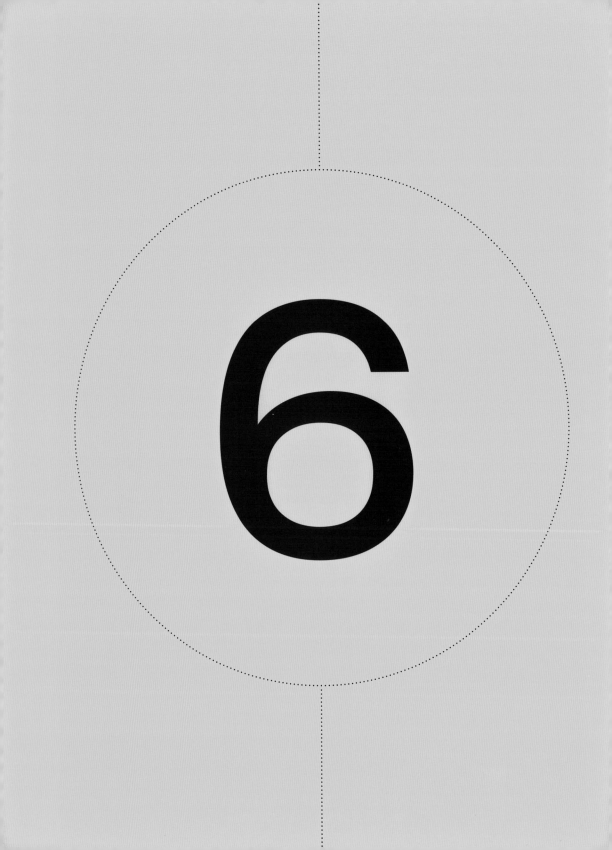

RECIPES

Before we get to the all-important conclusion (see pages 240-5), I've included 15 quick, easy and delicious recipes to get you started in the kitchen, or to add to your existing recipe bank. As I have touched on the importance of getting enough protein and fibre for overall health and losing weight, all recipes are high in protein or fibre, or both.

Whether it be breakfast, brunch, lunch or dinner, each of these recipes can slot into your own plan that you can build after reading this book. For example, if your calorie target is 2,000 calories per day for fat loss, you could enjoy my Folded bacon & egg tortilla for breakfast, my Meaty pizza for lunch and my Creamy breaded cod & chunky chips for dinner and still leave around 360 calories for other foods you enjoy. Perhaps a chocolate bar, some fruit and a biscuit? If you like these recipes, you should check out my second book, *Still Tasty*, which offers 100 reduced-calorie versions of your favourite, satisfying meals.

I love seeing you all post what you cook on Instagram. Please be sure to tag me and let me know how much you enjoy these recipes! Bon appetit!

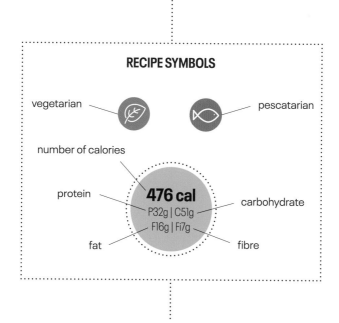

RECIPE SYMBOLS

vegetarian

pescatarian

number of calories

protein

476 cal
P32g | C51g
F16g | Fi7g

carbohydrate

fat

fibre

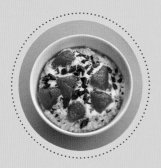

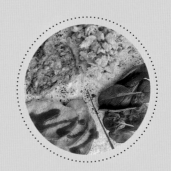

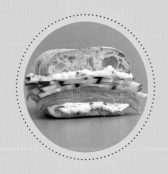

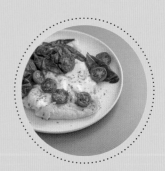

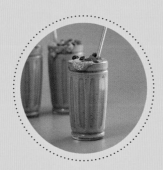

BREAKFAST
&
BRUNCH

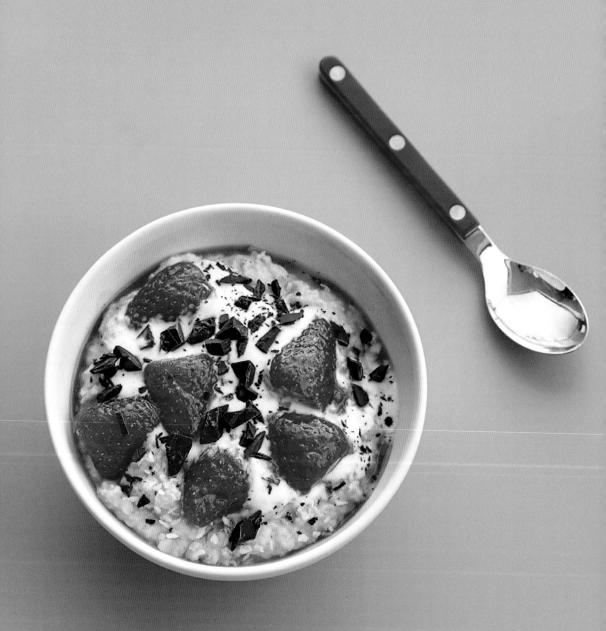

STRAWBERRY
& DARK CHOCOLATE
PORRIDGE

476 cal
P32g | C51g
F16g | Fi7g

HIGH
Protein
Fibre

Enjoy the delicious combination of strawberries and dark chocolate in this creamy, sweet porridge bowl. A happy way to start your day for under 500 calories.

TAKES 5 minutes
SERVES 1

50g rolled oats
250ml semi-skimmed milk
15g vanilla whey protein powder
Pinch of salt
2g desiccated coconut

20g 0% fat Greek yogurt
5 strawberries, hulled and chopped
1 square of 70% dark chocolate, broken into shards

Pour the oats and milk into a medium saucepan and set over a low–medium heat. Stir with wooden spoon for 4–5 minutes until the oats combine with the milk to become creamy. Keep stirring to avoid the porridge sticking to the bottom of the pan.

Once cooked, pour the porridge into a serving bowl and add the vanilla whey protein powder and salt. Stir in with a spoon until evenly combined.

Top the porridge with the desiccated coconut and yogurt. Squash the strawberries slightly and arrange over the top along with the dark chocolate and serve.

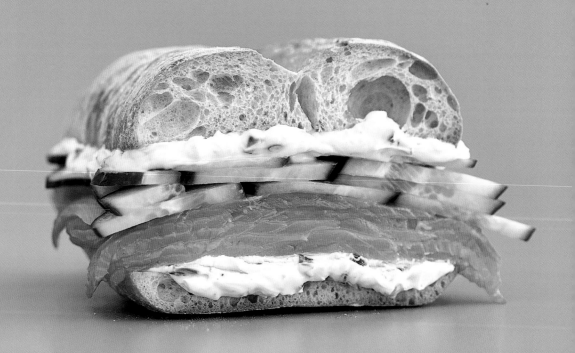

SMOKED SALMON
& CREAM CHEESE CIABATTA

522cal
P36g | C45g
F22g

Whether you're in a hurry or fancy something fast, look no further than this recipe! Enjoy crispy, soft-centred ciabatta, nutritious high-protein smoked salmon and cream cheese. You won't find this one on boring meal plans. Enjoy!

HIGH
Protein
Omega 3

....

TAKES 5 minutes
SERVES 1

....

100g ciabatta, halved
50g light cream cheese
3 chives, chopped
100g smoked salmon

10cm cucumber, halved and sliced
Juice of ¼ lemon
Black pepper

....

Toast both halves of the ciabatta.

Add the cream cheese, chives and some black pepper to a small bowl and mix with a spoon until well combined.

Spread both pieces of ciabatta with the cream cheese mixture. Top the bottom half with the smoked salmon and cucumber before gently squeezing over the lemon juice. Top with the top half of ciabatta and serve.

ON-THE-GO
BREAKFAST SMOOTHIE

537cal
P37g | C59g
F17g | Fi17g

HIGH
Protein
Fibre

If you have no time in the morning, you can still consume a balanced meal. Ready in just a couple of minutes, you can take this smoothie with you to drink on the way to work, setting you up with protein and micronutrients early in the day.

TAKES 2 minutes
SERVES 1

30g rolled oats
200ml almond milk
1 banana, sliced
30g chocolate whey protein powder
50g frozen raspberries

50g frozen blueberries
10g milled flaxseed,
  plus extra to serve
A few fresh berries, to serve

Add all the ingredients to a blender and blend until smooth.

Pour into a flask, top with a sprinkling of flaxseed and a few fresh berries and take with you to enjoy on the go.

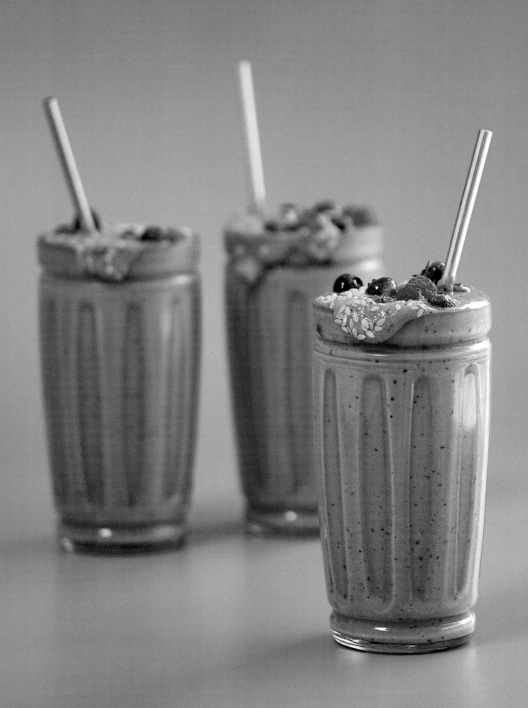

FOLDED BACON & EGG
BREAKFAST TORTILLA

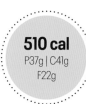

510 cal
P37g | C41g
F22g

HIGH
Protein

Perhaps you previously believed bacon and eggs were unhealthy. The good news is that this isn't the case. This recipe is packed with micronutrients and protein, ensuring it is both beneficial and delicious. Given bacon isn't something you want to eat every day, I recommend making this one once or twice a week – that way, you'll enjoy it even more!

TAKES 15 minutes
SERVES 1

Preheat the grill to high.

Add the bacon medallions to a foil-lined baking tray and grill for 5 minutes on each side.

While the bacon is grilling, crack the eggs into a small bowl and beat with a fork until smooth. Add the eggs to a small frying pan over a low heat. Scramble with a spatula for 4–6 minutes until cooked.

Add the avocado and lime juice to a small bowl, season with salt and pepper and mix together with a fork until well combined.

With a sharp knife, cut a line from the centre of the wrap to 6 o'clock. Add the grilled bacon medallions, mashed avocado, scrambled eggs and spinach separately on to the four quarters of the wrap, working clockwise from 6 o'clock. Top with the ketchup.

Fold the wrap in half, and then in half again to make a triangular sealed wrap.

Finally, add the folded wrap to a frying pan and cook for 1 minute on each side to crispen. Serve.

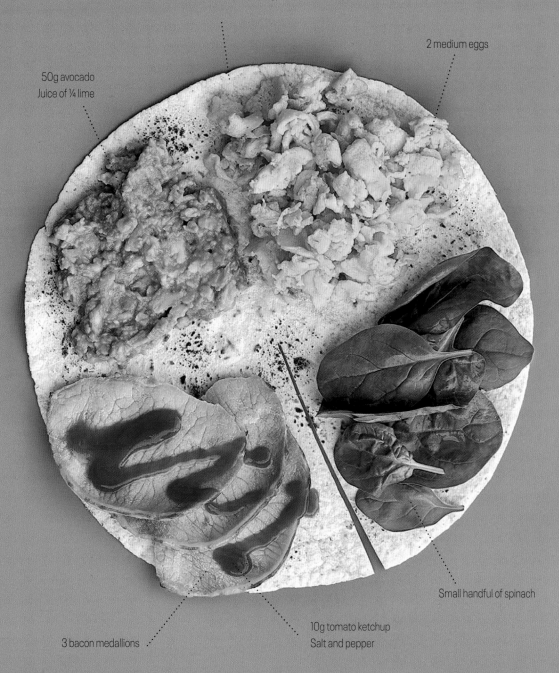

1 plain tortilla wrap (60g)

2 medium eggs

50g avocado
Juice of ¼ lime

Small handful of spinach

3 bacon medallions

10g tomato ketchup
Salt and pepper

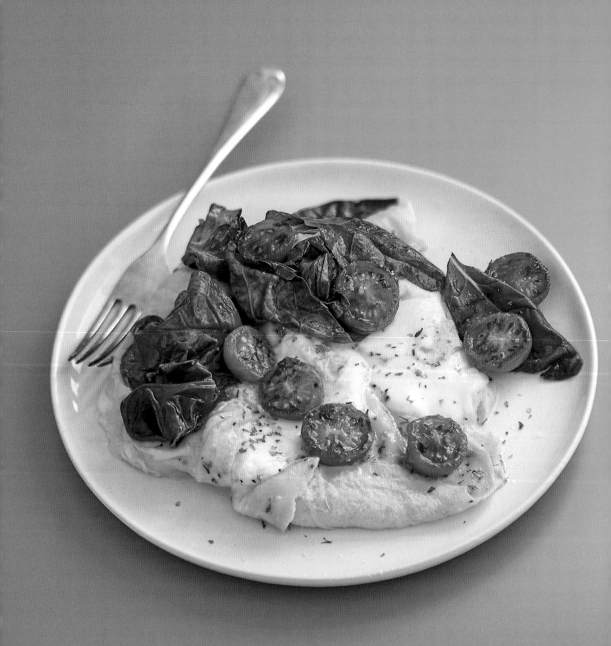

LOADED SPINACH, TOMATO & MOZZARELLA
FOLDED EGGS

432 cal
P33g | C3g
F32g

HIGH
Protein

A quick and easy breakfast packed with protein, micronutrients and flavour. Yes, you can eat this soon as you wake up!

TAKES 10 minutes
SERVES 1

5ml olive oil
3 medium eggs
Small handful of spinach
4 cherry tomatoes, halved

75g fresh mozzarella, sliced
½ tsp dried oregano
Salt and pepper

Add the olive oil to a medium frying pan over a medium–high heat.

Crack the eggs into a small bowl and beat with a fork until smooth. Pour the eggs into the frying pan and cook for 3–4 minutes, gently folding the eggs and moving the uncooked mixture to the middle of the pan until it's just set. Top with the spinach, cherry tomatoes and mozzarella and cook for a further 2–3 minutes over a low heat.

Slide the folded eggs from the frying pan on to a serving dish and season with salt, black pepper and the dried oregano. Serve.

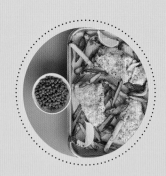

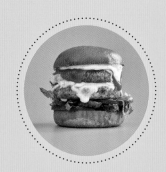

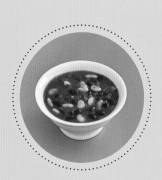

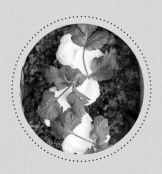

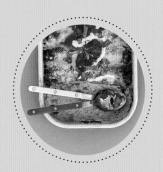

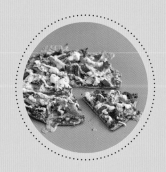

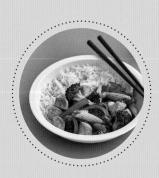

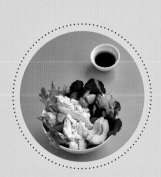

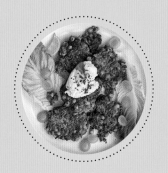

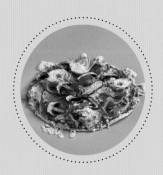

LUNCH
&
DINNER

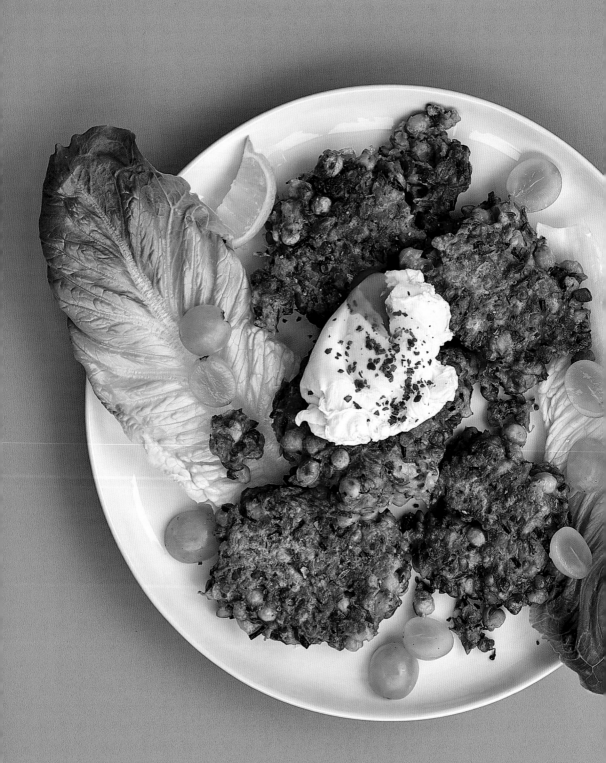

CHICKPEA & LENTIL FRITTERS
with a poached egg

518 cal
P28g | C70g
F14g | Fi22g

If you're looking for a high-fibre recipe, look no further than these crispy chickpea and lentil fritters. Adding a poached egg also boosts protein by 25 per cent! The combination of fibre and protein is not only great for your gut health but will also help you feel fuller for longer.

HIGH
Fibre

TAKES 10 minutes
SERVES 1

1 egg
Pinch of chilli flakes

For the fritters
150g cooked green lentils, drained
150g cooked chickpeas, drained
½ red onion, finely chopped
30g plain flour
Juice of ¼ lemon
Small handful of flat-leaf parsley, finely chopped

Small handful of chives, finely chopped
½ tsp dried Italian herbs
5ml olive oil
Salt and pepper

For the salad
3 leaves of romaine lettuce
7.5cm piece of cucumber, chopped
5 seedless green grapes, halved

Add all the fritter ingredients, except the olive oil, to a large bowl and mash with a potato masher until slightly lumpy.

Set a medium frying pan over a medium heat and add the olive oil. Add 2 tablespoons of fritter mixture to the pan, press down with a spatula and cook for 3–5 minutes on each side until golden. Repeat with the remaining mixture – you should have 4–5 fritters in total.

Half-fill a separate, small saucepan with water and bring to a simmer. Crack in the egg and poach for 3–4 minutes, then remove with a skimmer or slotted serving spoon.

Arrange the side salad on a serving plate before topping with the crispy fritters and poached egg. Scatter with the chilli flakes and serve.

EASY CHICKEN
& FETA SALAD

564 cal
P58g | C29g
F24g | Fi8g

If you're stuck for a flavoursome lunchtime feast, look no further than this delicious salad. Eating such an abundance of nutrients in one sitting leaves you able to enjoy that cookie or chocolate bar later on if you wish.

HIGH
Protein
Fibre

TAKES 5 minutes
SERVES 1

200g cooked chicken breast, sliced

For the dressing
5ml olive oil
10ml balsamic vinegar

1 medium pear, cored and chopped

5 cherry tomatoes, halved

Large handful of salad leaves

15cm piece of cucumber, chopped

Juice of ½ lime
Salt and pepper

Add all the salad ingredients to a large salad bowl and toss thoroughly to combine.

Combine the olive oil and balsamic vinegar for the dressing in a small bowl and mix with a spoon until completely dark. Add to the salad, tossing until thoroughly mixed in. Serve.

50g avocado, sliced

30g feta cheese, cubed

CAPRICCIOSA
PIZZA

Enjoy the authentic flavours and textures of this classic pizza, saving a huge number of calories by simply swapping a traditional pizza base for a tortilla wrap and regular Cheddar for a reduced-fat version. It tastes just as good and still provides many nutrients, as well as 33g protein, and all for under 500 calories.

TAKES 10 minutes
SERVES 1

Preheat the oven to 200°C.

To make the pizza sauce, combine the tomato purée, water and dried Italian herbs in a small bowl. Season with salt and pepper and mix until smooth, then spread evenly over the tortilla.

Transfer the tortilla to a pizza dish, then scatter over the toppings and bake for 5–7 minutes. Serve.

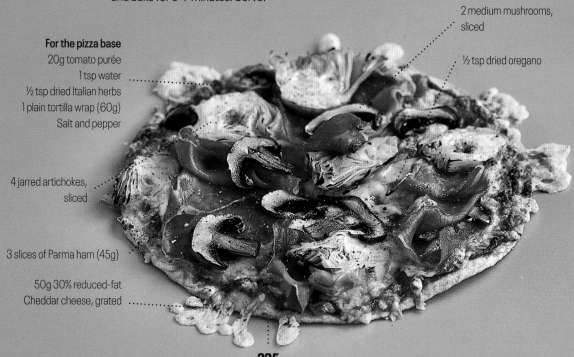

2 medium mushrooms, sliced

½ tsp dried oregano

For the pizza base
20g tomato purée
1 tsp water
½ tsp dried Italian herbs
1 plain tortilla wrap (60g)
Salt and pepper

4 jarred artichokes, sliced

3 slices of Parma ham (45g)

50g 30% reduced-fat Cheddar cheese, grated

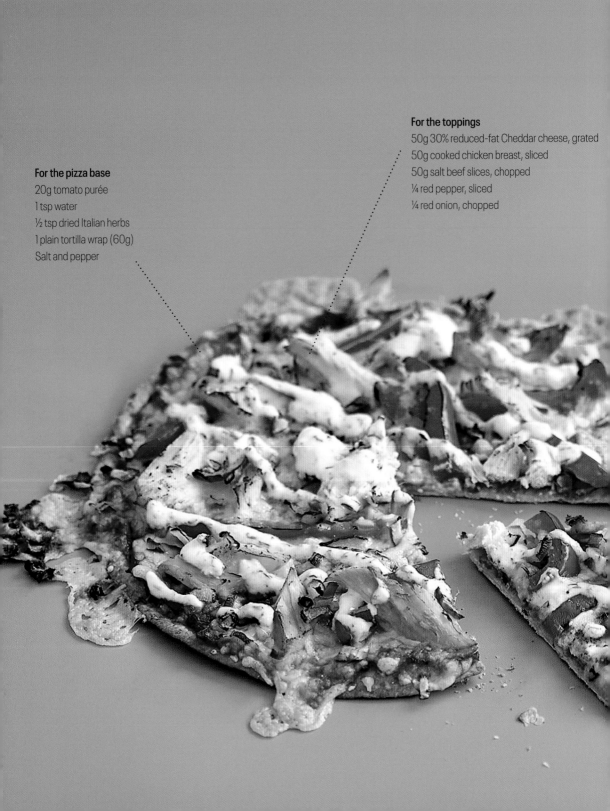

For the pizza base

20g tomato purée
1 tsp water
½ tsp dried Italian herbs
1 plain tortilla wrap (60g)
Salt and pepper

For the toppings

50g 30% reduced-fat Cheddar cheese, grated
50g cooked chicken breast, sliced
50g salt beef slices, chopped
¼ red pepper, sliced
¼ red onion, chopped

THE MEATY
PIZZA

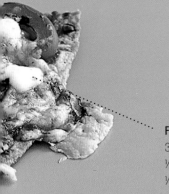

542 cal
P50g | C45g
F18g

HIGH
Protein

If you need to play catch up with protein, this delicious, meaty pizza has a whopping 50g. Ready in just 10 minutes, enjoy the succulent toppings, crispy base and creamy dip. It may be on a par with your favourite takeaway pizza, but crucially it's half the calories, helping you towards your weight-loss goal.

TAKES 10 minutes
SERVES 1

Preheat the oven to 200°C.

To make the pizza sauce, combine the tomato purée, water and dried Italian herbs in a small bowl. Season with salt and pepper and mix until smooth, then spread evenly over the tortilla.

Transfer the tortilla to a pizza dish, then scatter over the toppings and bake for 5–7 minutes.

Mix the Greek yogurt, garlic powder and oregano together in a small bowl until evenly combined. Drizzle over the cooked pizza and serve.

For the garlic dip
30g 0% fat Greek yogurt
½ tsp garlic powder
½ tsp dried oregano

CREAMY BREADED COD
& CHUNKY CHIPS

585 cal
P55g | C71g
F9g | Fi11g

Fish and chips is usually deemed off-limits for those who want to lose weight. This is because deep-frying food increases calories considerably, so by oven-cooking the ingredients, you can save hundreds of calories and enjoy the same succulent fish and crispy chips. By all means keep enjoying your favourite takeaway, but if you want to eat fish and chips regularly, this high-protein, nutrient-dense, fibre-rich recipe ticks all the boxes for balance and enjoyment for around half the calories.

HIGH
Protein
Fibre

TAKES 30 minutes
SERVES 2

250g potatoes, washed	20g dried breadcrumbs
5ml olive oil	100g frozen peas
30g 0% fat Greek yogurt	2g butter
10g light cream cheese	1 tsp hot sauce
3 chives, chopped	20g tomato ketchup
½ tsp garlic powder	A few lemon wedges
175g skinless cod fillet	Salt

Preheat the oven to 180°C.

Chop the potatoes into chunky chips, then add to a medium bowl with the olive oil and a pinch of salt. Mix with your hands until the chips are coated in the oil, then add to a lined baking tray. Bake for 25 minutes, shaking and turning after 15 minutes.

Add the Greek yogurt, cream cheese, chives and garlic powder to a small bowl and mix until smooth. Then spread evenly over the top of the cod.

Transfer the cod to a lined baking tray, then evenly scatter over the breadcrumbs, ensuring the creamy filling is covered. Bake for 15–20 minutes until the coating is golden brown.

Add the peas to a saucepan of boiling water and simmer for 2 minutes, then drain. Add the butter and hot sauce to the cooked peas, quickly stir, then transfer to a serving plate with the breaded cod, chunky chips, ketchup and a wedge of lemon.

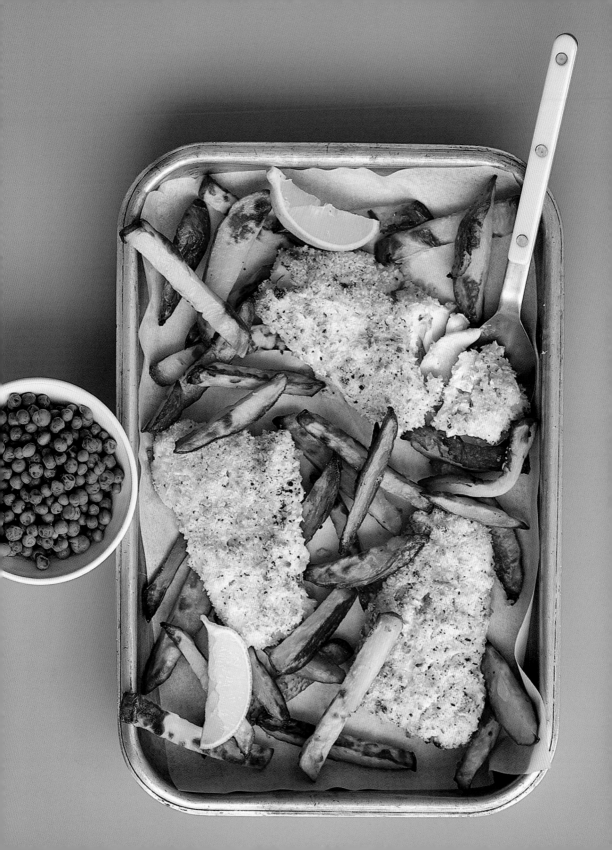

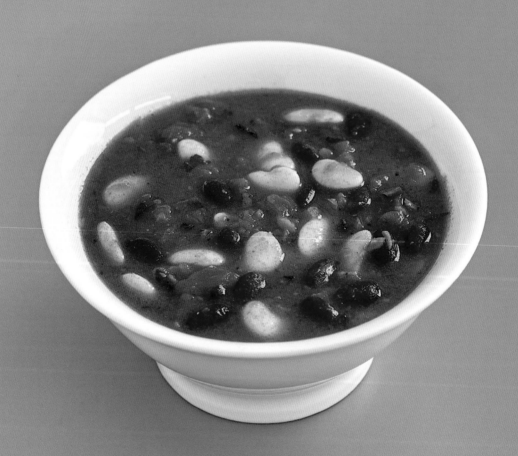

Any remaining portions
are perfect for freezing
or will keep in the fridge
for 2–3 days.

BEAN STEW

This veggie dish is easy, versatile and packed with a load of nutrients and fibre. Regularly including this tasty recipe in your diet will allow you to enjoy those meals out all the more, knowing you have struck the perfect balance of eating enough nutrients and enjoying less-nutritious foods in moderation.

362 cal
P21g | C47g
F10g | Fi22g

HIGH
Fibre

TAKES 15 minutes
SERVES 2

5ml olive oil
1 onion, chopped
4 garlic cloves, finely chopped
400g can chopped tomatoes
250g red kidney beans, drained
250g butter beans, drained
1½ tbsp smoked paprika

50g reduced-fat red pesto
Juice of ½ lemon
½ vegetable stock cube
100ml boiling water
2 tbsp finely chopped coriander
Salt and pepper

Set a large saucepan over a medium heat, then add the olive oil, onion and garlic. Cook for 2 minutes until they begin to soften and brown.

Add the chopped tomatoes, both beans and 1 tablespoon of smoked paprika and season with salt and pepper. Cook for a further 5 minutes until the mixture begins to bubble.

Reduce the heat, stir in the pesto, remaining smoked paprika, lemon juice, stock cube and boiling water and simmer for a further 5 minutes, stirring regularly. Stir through the coriander and serve.

TURKEY DOUBLE
CHEESEBURGER

594 cal
P73g | C35g
F18g

HIGH
Protein

If you struggle to hit your protein targets, this burger is for you. Enjoy all the traditional burger flavours but save calories by using turkey breast mince and reduced-fat cheese along with delicious toppings all in a brioche bun.

TAKES 20 minutes
SERVES 1

225g turkey breast mince
5ml olive oil
¼ onion, finely chopped
1 garlic clove, crushed
1 tsp dried oregano
1 tsp paprika
2 slices of reduced-fat Cheddar
cheese (50g)
5g low-fat mayonnaise

1 gherkin, thinly sliced
2 red onion rings
1 lettuce leaf
1 medium brioche bun (55g),
sliced in half
15g tomato ketchup
Salt and pepper

Preheat the grill to high.

Add the turkey mince, olive oil, onion, garlic, oregano and paprika to a large mixing bowl and season with salt and pepper. Mix thoroughly with your hands and form two evenly-sized meatballs. Transfer to a foil-lined baking dish and press down into two 2cm-thick burger patties. Grill for 7–8 minutes on each side until golden. Top each burger with a cheese slice for the last minute of grilling.

Add the mayonnaise, gherkin, red onion rings and lettuce to the bottom half of the brioche bun, followed by the turkey cheeseburgers. Top with the ketchup and the other half of the bun. Serve.

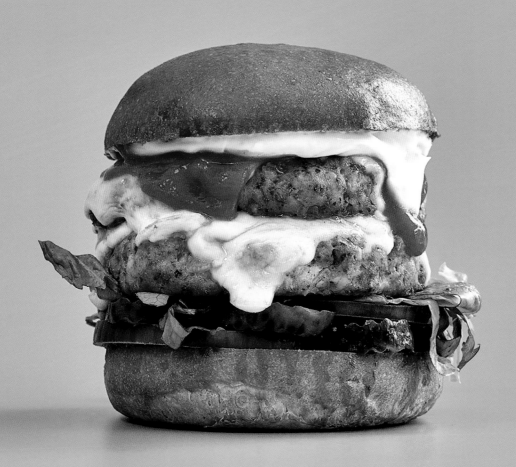

TERIYAKI
CHICKEN

443 cal
P45g | C50g
F7g

HIGH
Protein

If you're looking to increase your vegetable intake, look no further than this easy, delicious 15-minute chicken teriyaki. It's high in protein, oozing with nutrients and includes tasty rice. All for under 450 calories per portion.

TAKES 10 minutes
SERVES 2

5ml olive oil
1 red onion, finely chopped
3 garlic cloves, finely chopped
1 teaspoon peeled and chopped fresh ginger
300g skinless chicken breast, chopped
60ml teriyaki sauce

20ml light soy sauce
½ red pepper, chopped
5 baby corn, chopped
Small handful of green beans, chopped
250g pre-cooked microwave basmati rice

Set a medium pan over a medium heat, then add the olive oil, onion, garlic and ginger. Cook for 2 minutes until they begin to soften and brown.

Add the chicken and cook for 2 minutes until sealed.

Now add the teriyaki and soy sauces, pepper, baby corn and green beans, reduce the heat and cook for a further 7–8 minutes, stirring regularly.

Heat the basmati rice as per the packet instructions, then add to a serving dish with the teriyaki chicken. Serve.

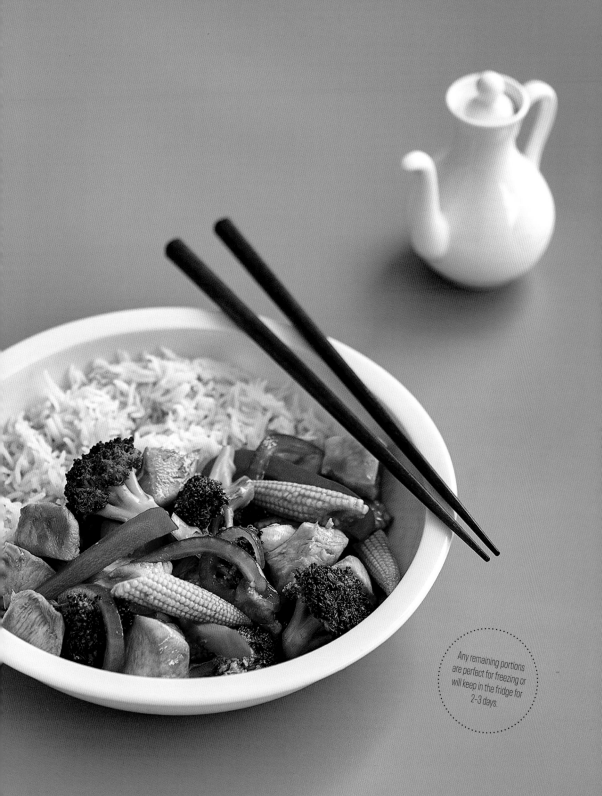

Any remaining portions are perfect for freezing or will keep in the fridge for 2–3 days.

BEEF
ENCHILADAS

577 cal
P48g | C58g
F17g

HIGH
Protein

This recipe is a real crowd-pleaser and ideal for feeding a gathering of family or friends. By swapping regular beef mince for 5% fat beef mince and regular Cheddar for a reduced-fat variety, you can enjoy the same flavours, but eat fewer calories to help achieve your weight-loss goal.

TAKES 25 minutes
SERVES 4

5ml olive oil
500g 5% fat beef mince
1 onion, chopped
4 garlic cloves, finely chopped
1 tbsp ground cumin
400g can chopped tomatoes
1 red pepper, deseeded and sliced
100g black beans, drained

1 tbsp chilli paste
10 x sprays olive oil cooking spray
8 x 40g corn tortilla wraps
150g 50% reduced-fat Cheddar
50g mild salsa
30g crème fraîche
A handful of coriander, chopped

Set a large frying pan over a medium heat, then add the olive oil, beef mince, onion, garlic and cumin. Cook for 3 minutes, breaking up the mince with a spatula.

Add the chopped tomatoes, red pepper, black beans and chilli paste and stir well. Cover with a lid and simmer for 10 minutes.

Preheat the oven to 200°C and grease a baking dish with the spray oil and kitchen paper.

Add the tortillas to the prepared dish and divide the beef sauce between the tortillas before rolling up and fitting next to each other tightly.

Scatter the Cheddar and salsa over the tortillas and bake for 8–10 minutes until the cheese is bubbling.

Remove from the oven, top with the crème fraîche and coriander. Serve.

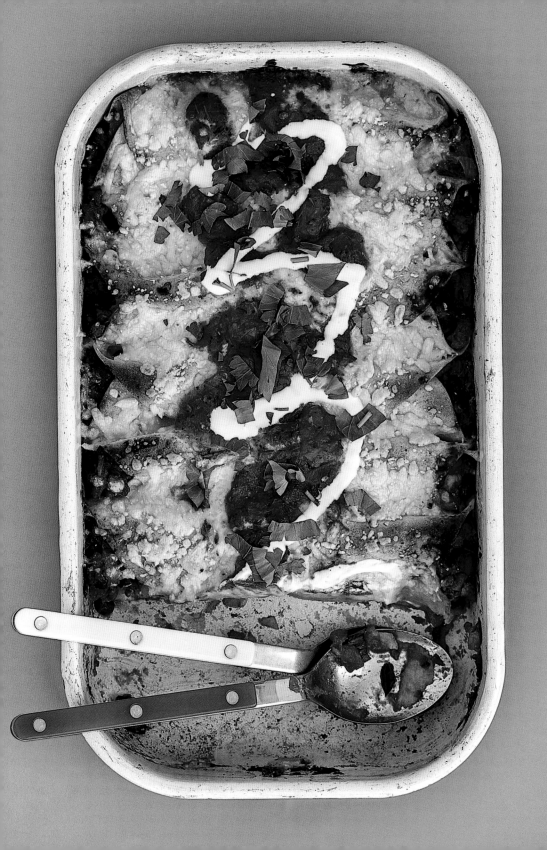

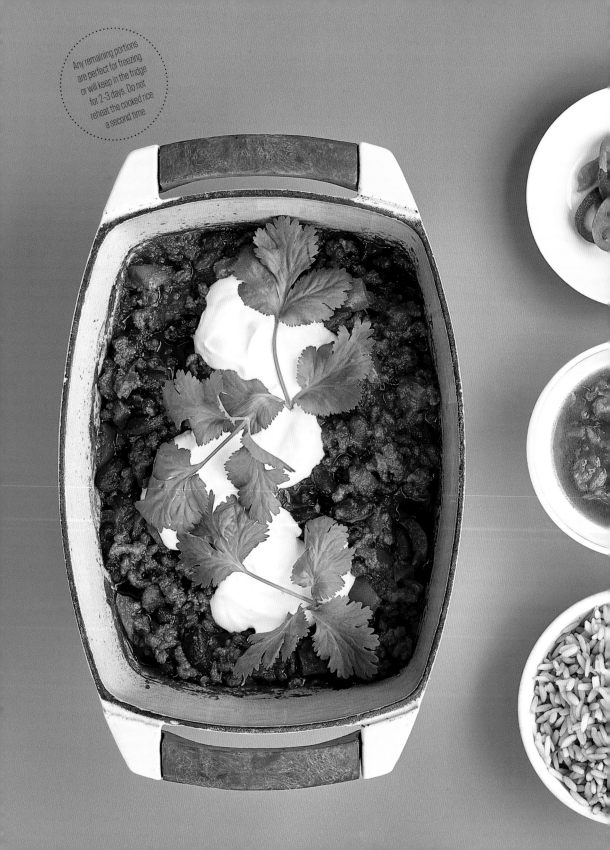

Any remaining portions are perfect for freezing or will keep in the fridge for 2–3 days. Do not reheat the cooked rice a second time.

CHILLI CON CARNE

This classic recipe is ideal for feeding your family or batch cooking and freezing. Enjoy fantastic flavours knowing you're eating a high amount of protein, fibre and micronutrients on a bed of delicious rice – which is absolutely allowed.

per portion with 125g brown rice

497 cal
P42g | C62g
F9g | Fi15g

HIGH
Protein
Fibre

TAKES 20 minutes
SERVES 4

5ml olive oil
1 large onion, chopped
4 garlic cloves, finely chopped
1 tbsp ground cumin
500g 5% fat beef mince
400g can chopped tomatoes
1 red pepper, deseeded and chopped
20g tomato purée
1 tsp smoked paprika
1 tsp light brown sugar
400g can of red kidney beans, drained

30g mild salsa
Salt and pepper
500g pre-cooked microwave brown rice

To serve
100g 0% fat Greek yogurt
Sprigs of fresh coriander
Sliced jalapeños (optional)

Heat a large frying pan over a medium heat, then add the olive oil, onion, garlic and cumin. Cook for 3 minutes until they begin to soften and brown.

Add the beef mince and cook for a further 3 minutes, breaking it up with a spatula until it begins to brown.

Reduce the heat, then add the chopped tomatoes, red pepper, tomato purée, smoked paprika, brown sugar and red kidney beans. Simmer for 7–8 minutes, stirring regularly.

Stir in the salsa and season with salt and black pepper. Cook for a further 2 minutes.

Add the pre-cooked brown rice to a microwavable dish and heat as per the packet instructions, then transfer to a serving dish along with the chilli con carne. Serve with a dollop of yogurt, some sprigs of coriander and sliced jalapeños, if you like.

CONCLUSION

Achieving lasting weight loss is not the result of sticking to a special diet, the latest fat-loss craze or regimented meal plans. It is determined by your mindset and the decisions you make over time. There's no need to demand excellence of yourself.

Each section of this book can help you to understand that losing weight for good and consuming a healthful diet can be simple, flexible and enjoyable.

1

You need a calorie deficit to lose weight, but you don't need to be perfect.

You need to make sure that the deficit is sustainable and flexible so you can stick to it for long periods of time. Remember, you are allowed to have a rich and fulfilling life outside of attempting to lose weight. Calorie counting can be great tool, keeping you informed on how your decisions might impact your goal. Increasing protein and fibre help you feel fuller and are easy adjustments that can make a huge difference over time. Finding bargains in the form of high-volume low-calorie foods is a great way to cut calories without feeling hungry. These tweaks to your existing diet set you up for something that is achievable and allow you to focus on all aspects of your life without any upheaval. This is the first step to trusting yourself to take control of your diet on your own terms.

2

There are no good or bad foods.

Arming yourself with this sentence can change your life. One doughnut does not make you fat or unhealthy, your overall diet across the days, weeks, months, years and decades of your life defines how healthy you are. Banning or restricting your favourite foods is nonsensical and will only make you want them more, which could mean trouble down the line. Removing morals from food allows us to see them for what they really are, free from baseless fearmongering, or unnecessary praise. The quality of the food you eat is important. For optimal health, we should base our diets on nutritious foods and make sure we eat enough protein, fibre and micronutrients. Whole foods like fruit, vegetables, lean meat, fish, beans and grains also fill us up for longer, meaning they are more likely to aid our fat loss efforts, too. But including less-nutritious foods we love now and again won't undo the healthful benefits we have already obtained. The idea that eating food containing chemicals, artificial ingredients and preservatives will poison us, or will make us fat or sick, is completely baseless. When asking for evidence to back up these claims, there simply isn't any. You don't deserve to feel guilty when you eat, and it turns out that there's no logical reason why you should either.

3

Don't get sucked in by media misinformation and diet tribes - look at the evidence instead.

Whether it be low carb, keto, eliminating sugar, intermittent fasting or slimming clubs, the science shows none of these diets are necessary for optimizing weight loss or overall health. Extreme factions of these diet camps continue to push their agendas with seemingly convincing, albeit flawed arguments. Decluttering your mind from misinformation allows you to separate truth from half-truth. It can be the difference between being led down the path to a miserable, unfulfilling diet you don't need and can't stick to, and enjoying a rich, fulfilling diet that supports your mental health.

4

Making small, simple changes and striving for 1 per cent improvements in your habits makes losing weight easier and, over time, compounds to create huge results.

By gradually planting your roots and expanding your branches, you are building a diet and lifestyle that cannot fall down. Enjoying the rewards of gradual change alongside getting everything you want out of your life is a sure-fire way to confidently remove the temptation of quick-fix diets that cause upheaval and can ruin your relationship with food and yourself.

5

Weight loss isn't something you can simply buy, order or demand instantly.

It is entirely dependent on averages over time. You don't need to lose vast amounts of weight to be successful. In fact, going slow will likely result in you going faster in the end; simply because you kept going and treated yourself well. You don't need perfection, willpower and resilience, and weight loss doesn't have to be a steep mountain you have to climb. You just need to be average, have your own motivation and a method you enjoy. Stay in tune with your emotional momentum and remember that at times when it may seem like you're getting nowhere, success may be just around the corner. You are allowed to enjoy yourself today because there is always tomorrow.

Losing weight without losing your mind means focusing on the processes, not the outcome. Despite all the noise, you already have a diet, and with evidence-based science, food you enjoy, simple changes and gradual improvements, you can plant your roots and gradually expand your branches to build a diet and lifestyle that is robust, supports your health, is full of joy and lasts forever.

NOTES

1   Nicklas JM, Huskey KW, Davis RB, Wee CC, 'Successful weight loss among obese U.S. adults', *Am J Prev Med* (2012); 42(5):481-485. doi:10.1016/j.amepre.2012.01.005.

2   Hall KD, Guo J, 'Obesity Energetics: Body Weight Regulation and the Effects of Diet Composition', *Gastroenterology* (2017); 152(7): 1718-1727.e3. doi:10.1053/j.gastro.2017.01.052.

3   Feehan LM, Geldman J, Sayre EC, *et al.*, 'Accuracy of Fitbit Devices: Systematic Review and Narrative Syntheses of Quantitative Data', *JMIR Mhealth Uhealth* (2018); 6(8): e10527. Published 2018 Aug 9. doi:10.2196/10527.

4   Nuss KJ, Thomson EA, Courtney JB, Comstock A, Reinwald S, Blake S, E R, Tracy BL, Li K, 'Assessment of Accuracy of Overall Energy Expenditure Measurements for the Fitbit Charge HR 2 and Apple Watch', *Am J Health Behav* (2019 May 1); 43(3): 498-505. doi: 10.5993/AJHB.43.3.5. PMID: 31046881.

5   Hu MX, Turner D, Generaal E, Bos D, Ikram MK, Ikram MA, Cuijpers P, Penninx BWJH, 'Exercise interventions for the prevention of depression: a systematic review of meta-analyses', *BMC Public Health* (2020 Aug 18); 20(1): 1255. doi: 10.1186/s12889-020-09323-y. PMID: 32811468; PMCID: PMC7436997.

6   von Loeffelholz C, Birkenfeld A, 'The Role of Non-exercise Activity Thermogenesis in Human Obesity'. [Updated 2018 Apr 9].

7   Lichtman SW, Pisarska K, Berman ER, Pestone M, Dowling H, Offenbacher E, Weisel H, Heshka S, Matthews DE, Heymsfield SB, 'Discrepancy between self-reported and actual caloric intake and exercise in obese subjects', *N Engl J Med* (1992 Dec 31); 327(27): 1893-8. doi: 10.1056/NEJM199212313272701. PMID: 1454084.

8   Polivy J, 'Psychological consequences of food restriction', *J Am Diet Assoc* (1996 Jun); 96(6): 589-92; quiz 593-4. doi: 10.1016/S0002-8223(96)00161-7. PMID: 8655907.

9   FAO, IFAD, UNICEF, WFP and WHO. 2021, 'The State of Food Security and Nutrition in the World 2021. Transforming food systems for food security, improved nutrition and affordable healthy diets for all', Rome, FAO.

10   Nigg JT, Lewis K, Edinger T, Falk M, 'Meta-analysis of attention-deficit/hyperactivity disorder or attention-deficit/hyperactivity disorder symptoms, restriction diet, and synthetic food color additives', *J Am Acad Child Adolesc Psychiatry* (2012); 51(1): 86-97. e8. doi:10.1016/j.jaac.2011.10.015.

11   Bastaki M, Farrell T, Bhusari S, Bi X, Scrafford C, 'Estimated daily intake and safety of FD&C food-colour additives in the US population', *Food Addit Contam Part A Chem Anal Control Expo Risk Assess* (2017 Jun); 34(6): 891-904. DOI: 10.1080/19440049.2017.1308018. Epub 2017 Apr 19. Erratum in *Food Addit Contam Part A Chem Anal Control Expo Risk Assess* (2017 Jun); 34(6):x. PMID: 28332449.

12   Boeing H, Bechthold A, Bub A, Ellinger S, Haller D, Kroke A, Leschik-Bonnet E, Müller MJ, Oberritter H, Schulze M, Stehle P, Watzl B, 'Critical review: vegetables and fruit in the prevention of chronic diseases', *Eur J Nutr* (2012 Sep); 51(6): 637-63. doi: 10.1007/s00394-012-0380-y. Epub 2012 Jun 9. PMID: 22684631; PMCID: PMC34193.

13   Arnotti K, Bamber M, 'Fruit and Vegetable Consumption in Overweight or Obese Individuals: A Meta-Analysis', *West J Nurs Res* (2020 Apr); 42(4): 306-314. doi: 10.1177/0193945919858699. Epub 2019 Jun 29. PMID: 31256714.

14   Gianfredi V, Salvatori T, Villarini M, Moretti M, Nucci D, Realdon S, 'Is dietary fibre truly protective against colon cancer? A systematic review and meta-analysis', *Int J Food Sci Nutr* (2018 Dec); 69(8): 904-915. doi: 10.1080/09637486.2018.1446917. Epub 2018 Mar 8. PMID: 29516760.

15   Holt SH, Miller JC, Petocz P, Farmakalidis E, 'A satiety index of common foods', *Eur J Clin Nutr* (1995 Sep); 49(9): 675-90. PMID: 7498104.

16   Leidy HJ, Todd CB, Zino AZ, Immel JE, Mukherjea R, Shafer RS, Ortinau LC, Braun M, 'Consuming High-Protein Soy Snacks Affects Appetite Control, Satiety, and Diet Quality in Young People and Influences Select Aspects of Mood and Cognition', *J Nutr* (2015 Jul); 145(7): 1614-22. doi: 10.3945/jn.115.212092. Epub 2015 May 20. PMID: 2599528.

17   Kim JE, O'Connor LE, Sands LP, Slebodnik MB, Campbell WW, 'Effects of dietary protein intake on body composition changes after weight loss in older adults: a systematic review and meta-analysis', *Nutr Rev* (2016 Mar); 74(3): 210-24. doi: 10.1093/nutrit/nuv065. Epub 2016 Feb 16. PMID: 26883880; PMCID: PMC48922.

18   Chen, X., Zhang, Z., Yang, H. *et al.*, 'Consumption of ultra-processed foods and health outcomes: a systematic review of epidemiological studies', *Nutr J* (2020) 19, 86.

19   Weiskirchen S, Weiskirchen R, 'Resveratrol: How Much Wine Do You Have to Drink to Stay Healthy?'. *Adv Nutr.* (2016); 7(4): 706-718. Published 2016 Jul 15. doi:10.3945/an.115.011627.

20 Toews I, Lohner S, Küllenberg de Gaudry D, Sommer H, Meerpohl JJ, 'Association between intake of non-sugar sweeteners and health outcomes: systematic review and meta-analyses of randomised and non-randomised controlled trials and observational studies' [published correction appears in *BMJ* (2019 Jan 15); 364: l156]. *BMJ*. (2019); 364: k4718. Published 2019 Jan 2. doi:10.1136/bmj.k4718.

21 Rogers PJ, Appleton KM, 'The effects of low-calorie sweeteners on energy intake and body weight: a systematic review and meta-analyses of sustained intervention studies', *Int J Obes* (Lond) (2021 Mar); 45(3): 464–478. doi: 10.1038/s41366-020-00704-2. Epub 2020 Nov 9. Erratum in: *Int J Obes* (Lond) (2021 May 27). PMID: 33168917.

22 Lasschuijt MP, Mars M, de Graaf C, Smeets PAM, 'Endocrine Cephalic Phase Responses to Food Cues: A Systematic Review', *Adv Nutr* (2020 Sep 1); 11(5): 1364–1383. doi: 10.1093/advances/nmaa059. PMID: 32516803; PMCID: PMC7490153.

23 Santos NC, de Araujo LM, De Luca Canto G, Guerra ENS, Coelho MS, Borin MF, 'Metabolic effects of aspartame in adulthood: A systematic review and meta-analysis of randomized clinical trials', *Crit Rev Food Sci Nutr* (2018); 58(12): 2068–2081. doi: 10.1080/10408398.2017.1304358. Epub 2017 Aug 18. PMID: 28394643.

24 Ahmad SY, Friel J, Mackay D, 'The Effects of Non-Nutritive Artificial Sweeteners, Aspartame and Sucralose, on the Gut Microbiome in Healthy Adults: Secondary Outcomes of a Randomized Double-Blinded Crossover Clinical Trial', *Nutrients* (2020 Nov 6); 12(11): 3408. doi: 10.3390/nu12113408. PMID: 33171964; PMCID: PMC7694690.

25 Bordoni A, Danesi F, Dardevet D, Dupont D, Fernandez AS, Gille D, Nunes Dos Santos C, Pinto P, Re R, Rémond D, Shahar DR, Vergères G, 'Dairy products and inflammation: A review of the clinical evidence', *Crit Rev Food Sci Nutr* (2017 Aug 13); 57(12): 2497–2525. doi: 10.1080/10408398.2014.967385. PMID: 26287637.

26 Bordoni A, Danesi F, Dardevet D, Dupont D, Fernandez AS, Gille D, Nunes Dos Santos C, Pinto P, Re R, Rémond D, Shahar DR, Vergères G, 'Dairy products and inflammation: A review of the clinical evidence', *Crit Rev Food Sci Nutr* (2017 Aug 13); 57(12): 2497–2525. doi: 10.1080/10408398.2014.967385. PMID: 26287637.

27 Blazey T, Snyder AZ, Goyal MS, Vlassenko AG, Raichle ME, 'A systematic meta-analysis of oxygen-to-glucose and oxygen-to-carbohydrate ratios in the resting human brain', *PLOS One* (2018); 13(9): e0204242. doi:10.1371/journal.pone.0204242.

28 Schwingshackl L, Bogensberger B, Benčič A, Knüppel S, Boeing H, Hoffmann G, 'Effects of oils and solid fats on blood lipids: a systematic review and network meta-analysis', *J Lipid Res* (2018); 59(9): 1771–1782. doi:10.1194/jlr.P085522.

29 Clarke R, Frost C, Collins R, Appleby P, Peto R, 'Dietary lipids and blood cholesterol: quantitative meta-analysis of metabolic ward studies', *BMJ* (1997 Jan 11); 314(7074): 112–7. doi: 10.1136/bmj.314.7074.112. PMID: 9006469; PMCID: PMC2125600.

30 Hooper L, Martin N, Jimoh OF, Kirk C, Foster E, Abdelhamid AS, 'Reduction in saturated fat intake for cardiovascular disease', *Cochrane Database Syst Rev* (2020 Aug 21); 8(8): CD011737. doi: 10.1002/14651858.CD011737.pub3. PMID: 32827219; PMCID: PMC8092457.

31 https://foodinsight.org/wp-content/uploads/2018/05/2018-FHS-Report.pdf

32 https://foodinsight.org/wp-content/uploads/2020/06/IFIC-Food-and-Health-Survey-2020.pdf

33 Esteves de Oliveira FC, Pinheiro Volp AC, Alfenas RC, 'Impact of different protein sources in the glycemic and insulinemic responses', *Nutr Hosp* (2011 Jul-Aug); 26(4): 669–76. doi: 10.1590/S0212-16112011000400002. PMID: 22470009.

34 Manders RJ, Hansen D, Zorenc AH, Dendale P, Kloek J, Saris WH, van Loon LJ, 'Protein co-ingestion strongly increases postprandial insulin secretion in type 2 diabetes patients', *J Med Food* (2014 Jul); 17(7): 758–63. doi: 10.1089/jmf.2012.0294. Epub 2014 Mar 10. PMID: 24611935.

35 Hall KD, Chen KY, Guo J, Lam YY, Leibel RL, Mayer LE, Reitman ML, Rosenbaum M, Smith SR, Walsh BT, Ravussin E, 'Energy expenditure and body composition changes after an isocaloric ketogenic diet in overweight and obese men', *Am J Clin Nutr* (2016 Aug); 104(2): 324–33. doi: 10.3945/ajcn.116.133561. Epub 2016 Jul 6. PMID: 27385608; PMCID: PMC4962163.

36 Ashtary-Larky D, Bagheri R, Bavi H, Baker JS, Moro T, Mancin L, Paoli A, 'Ketogenic diets, physical activity, and body composition: A review', *Br J Nutr* (2021 Jul); 12: 1–68. doi: 10.1017/S0007114521002609. Epub ahead of print. PMID: 34250885.

37 Kempner W, Newborg BC, Peschel RL, Skyler JS, 'Treatment of massive obesity with rice/reduction diet program. An analysis of 106 patients with at least a 45-kg weight loss', *Arch Intern Med* (1975 Dec); 135(12): 1575–84. PMID: 1200726.

38 Hall KD, Guo J, 'Obesity Energetics: Body Weight Regulation and the Effects of Diet Composition', *Gastroenterology* (2017); 152(7): 1718–1727.e3. doi:10.1053/j.gastro.2017.01.052.

39 Te Morenga L, Mallard S, Mann J, 'Dietary sugars and body weight: systematic review and meta-analyses of randomised controlled trials and cohort studies', 2013. In: Database of Abstracts of Reviews of Effects (DARE): Quality-assessed Reviews [Internet]. York (UK): Centre for Reviews and Dissemination (UK); 1995-. Available from: https://www.ncbi.nlm.nih.gov/books/NBK116814/

40 Khan TA, Sievenpiper JL, 'Controversies about sugars: results from systematic reviews and meta-analyses on obesity, cardiometabolic disease and diabetes', *Eur J Nutr* (2016); 55(Suppl 2): 25–43. doi:10.1007/s00394-016-1345-3.

41 USDA Economic research service, CDC NHANES surveys.

42 USDA Economic research service, CDC NHANES surveys.

43 Lenoir M, Serre F, Cantin L, Ahmed SH, 'Intense sweetness surpasses cocaine reward', *PLOS One* (2007); 2(8): e698. doi:10.1371/journal.pone.0000698.

44 Schulte EM, Avena NM, Gearhardt AN, 'Which foods may be addictive? The roles of processing, fat content, and glycemic load', *PLOS One* (2015 Feb 18); 10(2): e0117959. doi: 10.1371/journal.pone.0117959. PMID: 25692302; PMCID: PMC4334652.

45 Rena R Wing, Suzanne Phelan, 'Long-term weight loss maintenance', *Am J Clin Nutr* (2005 Jul); 82(1): 222S–225S.

46 Cioffi I, Evangelista A, Ponzo V, *et al.*, 'Intermittent versus continuous energy restriction on weight loss and cardiometabolic outcomes: a systematic review and meta-analysis of randomized controlled trials', *J Transl Med* (2018); 16(1): 371. doi:10.1186/s12967-018-1748-4.

47 Bagheriya M, Butler AE, Barreto GE, Sahebkar A, 'The effect of fasting or calorie restriction on autophagy induction: A review of the literature', *Ageing Res Rev* (2018 Nov); 47: 183–197. doi: 10.1016/j.arr.2018.08.004. Epub 2018 Aug 30. PMID: 30172870.

48 Levine JA, Eberhardt NL, Jensen MD, 'Role of nonexercise activity thermogenesis in resistance to fat gain in humans', *Science* (1999 Jan 8); 283(5399): 212–4. doi: 10.1126/science.283.5399.212. PMID: 9880251.

49 'Archytas of Tarentum, Technology Museum of Thessaloniki, Macedonia, Greece', Tmth.edu.gr. Archived from the original on 2008-12-26. Retrieved 2013-05-30.

50 Wang X, Sparks JR, Bowyer KP, Youngstedt SD, 'Influence of sleep restriction on weight loss outcomes associated with caloric restriction', *Sleep* (2018 May 1); 41(5). doi: 10.1093/sleep/zsy027. PMID: 29438540.

51 Fothergill E, Guo J, Howard L, Kerns JC, Knuth ND, Brychta R, Chen KY, Skarulis MC, Walter M, Walter PJ, Hall KD, 'Persistent metabolic adaptation 6 years after "The Biggest Loser" competition', *Obesity* (2016 Aug); 24(8): 1612–9. doi: 10.1002/oby.21538. Epub 2016 May 2. PMID: 27136388; PMCID: PMC4989512.

52 Fothergill E, Guo J, Howard L, Kerns JC, Knuth ND, Brychta R, Chen KY, Skarulis MC, Walter M, Walter PJ, Hall KD, 'Persistent metabolic adaptation 6 years after "The Biggest Loser" competition', *Obesity* (2016 Aug); 24(8): 1612–9. doi: 10.1002/oby.21538. Epub 2016 May 2. PMID: 27136388; PMCID: PMC4989512.

53 https://www.scientificamerican.com/article/6-years-after-the-biggest-loser-metabolism-is-slower-and-weight-is-back-up/

54 Reba-Harrelson L, Von Holle A, Thornton LM, *et al.*, 'Features associated with diet pill use in individuals with eating disorders', *Eat Behav* (2008); 9(1): 73–81. doi:10.1016/j.eatbeh.2007.04.001.

55 Levinson JA, Sarda V, Sonneville K, Calzo JP, Ambwani S, Austin SB, 'Diet Pill and Laxative Use for Weight Control and Subsequent Incident Eating Disorder in US Young Women: 2001-2016', *Am J Public Health* (2020 Jan); 110(1): 109–111. doi: 10.2105/AJPH.2019.305390. Epub 2019 Nov 21. PMID: 31751147; PMCID: PMC6893330.

56 Hall KD, Kahan S, 'Maintenance of Lost Weight and Long-Term Management of Obesity', *Med Clin North Am* (2018); 102(1): 183–197. doi:10.1016/j.mcna.2017.08.012.

57 Perri MG, McAllister DA, Gange JJ, *et al.*, 'Effects of four maintenance programs on the long-term management of obesity', *J Consult Clin Psychol* (1988); 56(4): 529–534.

INDEX

ACKNOWLEDGEMENTS

I would firstly like to thank all of you for trusting me by purchasing this book, and my previous books too. I'd like to thank everyone at Ebury, Penguin Random House, especially Laura Higginson and Vicky Orchard. To Sophie Yamamoto, who has provided another wonderful book design, Hannah Pemberton, for her delicious photography of my recipes, and to my agent Jen, who has been paramount in getting my ideas published.

A special thanks goes to my family who continue to support me – thank you.

By the same author
Eat What You Like & Lose Weight For Life
Still Tasty

Ebury Press, an imprint of Ebury Publishing
20 Vauxhall Bridge Road
London SW1V 2SA

Ebury Press is part of the Penguin Random House group of companies
whose addresses can be found at global.penguinrandomhouse.com

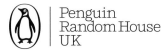

Text © Graeme Tomlinson 2022
Recipe photography by Hannah Pemberton © Ebury Press 2022
Additional photo credits: p.6 and back cover photograph: Matt Russell,
p.147 Akihito Yamamoto, Adobe stock: front cover © dzimin,
p.19 © Konovalov Pavel, p.21 © rashadashurov, p.51 © Oceloti,
p.101 © DKG1111, p.123&187 © barks, p.123 © SMUX, p.123 © warmworld,
p.144 © amine1976, p.144 © vectorplus, p.144 © Michal Hubka,
p.146 © Arcady, p.148-150 © Salamatik, p.150 © 3dwithlove,
p.150 © Mrson, p.150 © ylivdesign, p.191 © chrupka, p.191 ©
krissikunterbunt, p.198 © M-KOS, p.199 © dymentyd , p.199 © klamite

First published by Ebury Press in 2022
www.penguin.co.uk

A CIP catalogue record for this book is available
from the British Library

ISBN 978-1-52914-930-2

Designed by maru studio
Colour origination by Altaimage London
Printed and bound in Italy by L.E.G.O. S.p.A

The authorised representative in the EEA
is Penguin Random House Ireland,
Morrison Chambers, 32 Nassau Street,
Dublin D02 YH68.

Penguin Random House is committed to a sustainable future
for our business, our readers and our planet. This book
is made from Forest Stewardship Council® certified paper.

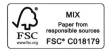

NOTE: The information in this book has been compiled by way of general guidance in
relation to the specific subjects addressed, but is not a substitute and not to be relied
on for medical, healthcare, pharmaceutical or other professional advice on specific
circumstances and in specific locations. Please consult your GP before changing,
stopping or starting any medical treatment. So far as the author is aware the information
given is correct and up to date as at September 2021. Practice, laws and regulations all
change, and the reader should obtain up to date professional advice on any such issues.
The author and publishers disclaim, as far as the law allows, any liability arising directly or
indirectly from the use, or misuse, of the information contained in this book.

'Yours is the best cookbook I've ever owned! (And I've got a few!) I love that I get to still eat carbs and I've managed to get rid of my stubborn stomach fat in a week (along with 2 other controlled meals and daily exercise).' Nicola, UK

'For the first time ever I'm actually enjoying a "diet" because I can still eat some of the things I like and lose weight.' Lee, UK

'You are the ONLY account I still allow myself to follow through my eating disorder recovery!' Angela, USA

'I bloody love your content!! Keep up the good work as it's really helped me and it's starting to help my girlfriend as well as I'm showing her. She sees food in a whole new light and it's so simple to understand.' Andrew, UK

'I came across your page a year or so ago and bought both your books. Loved how they were written so simply, and it was easy to understand why I wasn't losing weight. Six months ago I finally got my mental health in check and have now lost over 2.5 stone by calorie counting. I eat anything I want, whenever I want, just keep within my 1,800 daily allowance.' Beki, UK